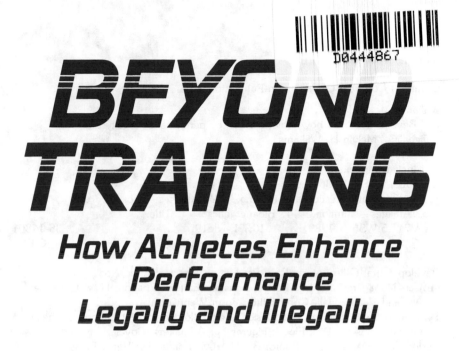

BEYOND TRAINING

How Athletes Enhance Performance Legally and Illegally

Melvin H. Williams, PhD

Director, Human Performance Laboratory
Old Dominion University

Leisure Press
Champaign, Illinois

Library of Congress Cataloging-in-Publication Data

Williams, Melvin H.
  Beyond training : how athletes enhance performance legally and
illegally / Melvin H. Williams.
    p.   cm.
  Includes index.
  ISBN 0-88011-336-7
    1. Physical education and training.   2. Athletes—Substance use.
  3. Athletes—Nutrition.   4. Bioenergetics.   I. Title.
  GV711.5.W55   1989   613.7'1—dc19   88-14801
                                                                CIP

Developmental Editor: Marie Roy; Production Director: Ernie Noa
Projects Manager: Janet Lea Peters; Assistant Editors: Phaedra Hise, Christine
Drews, and Valerie Hall; Copy Editor: John Wentworth;
Typesetter: Sandra Meier; Text Design: Keith Blomberg; Text Layout: Michelle
Baum; Cartoons by: Dick Flood; Figures by: Admakers; Cover
Design: Jack Davis; Cover Photo: Bill Morrow; Printed by: Versa Press

ISBN: 0-88011-336-7

Printed in the United States of America   10 9 8 7 6 5

Leisure Press
A Division of Human Kinetics Publishers
P.O. Box 5076, Champaign, IL 61825-5076
1-800-747-4457

Canada: Human Kinetics Publishers, P.O. Box 2503, Windsor, ON N8Y 4S2
1-800-465-7301 (in Canada only)

Europe: Human Kinetics Publishers (Europe) Ltd., P.O. Box IW14,
Leeds LS16 6TR, England
0532-781708

Australia: Human Kinetics Publishers, P.O. Box 80, Kingswood 5062, South Australia
618-374-0433

New Zealand: Human Kinetics Publishers, P.O. Box 105-231, Auckland 1
(09) 309-2259

Contents

List of Tables

Notice

The purpose of this book is to serve as a reference source only. The information provided is designed to help athletes make informed decisions regarding the use of special (ergogenic) aids as a means to improve performance in sport. The ethical, legal, and medical implications regarding the use of any ergogenic aid should be considered by all athletes prior to its use.

Preface

WHAT ARE THE ETHICS OF sport? According to the *Oxford English Dictionary*, the definition of *ethics* includes the following:

1. Moral principles of a particular school of thought
2. Rules of conduct recognized in certain associations
3. Moral principles by which an individual is guided

We can see that all three definitions are operational in sport. The ancient Greek ideal, that athletes should succeed through their own unaided effort, is a school of thought (definition 1) embraced by many athletes and organizations today, including the International Olympic Committee. Within this committee, certain associations, such as the International Amateur Cycling Federation, establish specific rules of conduct (definition 2) to promote athletes' adherence to the Greek ideal and to discourage them from obtaining unfair advantages. However, the athlete whose primary goal is to win at all costs may be guided by his or her own principles (definition 3) in an attempt to obtain that unfair advantage.

We have all heard the Olympic ideal paraphrased as "Do your best with what you've got." The "what you've got" originally referred to the athlete's natural athletic abilities, finely tuned through vigorous physical training with the guidance of a coach and trainer. However, more and more elite athletes participating in international competition are learning to modify their natural abilities with techniques above and beyond normal training in order to get an advantage—and not necessarily an unfair one—over their competitors. They are being assisted in these endeavors by a variety of sport scientists, including sport nutritionists, sport psychologists, sport physiologists, sport biomechanists, and even sport pharmacologists.

Many of these sport scientists are researching means to maximize human athletic potential. In the past 30 years we have seen a tremendous increase in the amount of research devoted to exercise and sport. Much of this research was conducted simply to understand the basic physiological, psychological, and biomechanical nature of athletic performance. Once this basic nature was determined, some investigators manipulated relevant variables in attempts to improve performance. For example, research has provided us with fairly good information regarding the basic physiological adjustments of the cardiovascular system to deliver oxygen to the muscle tissues during exercise. Some researchers have taken this information and developed ways to increase the oxygen delivery, which would be important to endurance athletes.

The special substances or treatments used in attempts to improve physiological, psychological, or biomechanical functions important to sport are usually known as *ergogenic aids*, for *ergogenic* means simply to increase the rate of work output. As shall be noted throughout the book, many of the ergogenic aids may be used to improve athletic performance in certain situations and may provide an athlete with a competitive advantage. Some ergogenic aids may confer a fair competitive advantage; others may be considered unfair because their use in sport has been banned.

I have had experience with ergogenic aids on several levels. As a college athlete I used nutritional ergogenic aids, such as protein supplements, in attempts to gain muscle mass for football. As a marathoner and ultramarathoner I have used a pharmacological ergogenic aid, caffeine, in attempts to improve endurance. As a coach at both the high school and college level I used psychological ergogenic aids in attempts to improve performance of my athletes (although I must admit that at the time I did not know them as psychological aids). As a sport scientist the focus of research in my laboratory over the past 20 years has been on ergogenic aids, including nutritional, pharmacological, psychological, and physiological aids.

In 1983 I was fortunate to be in a position to edit the book *Ergogenic Aids in Sport* for Human Kinetics Publishers. Some of the leading sport scientists in the United States contributed to the book, which was developed primarily for our peers—other sport scientists. In general, it was a rather technical review of the scientific literature regarding 13 different ergogenic aids.

Rainer Martens, the president of Human Kinetics, suggested to me that a book on ergogenic aids might have broader appeal if the presentation met the needs of all athletes involved in sport—not only the elite and college athletes and their coaches, but also the everyday athlete who wants to do his or her best in athletic competition, be it a local 10-kilometer road race, a minitriathlon, or any sport in which an athlete may benefit from the use of an appropriate ergogenic aid. This book has been written with that goal in mind.

Acknowledgments

I WOULD LIKE TO ACKNOWLEDGE deep gratitude to my many students and colleagues over the years who have participated in our research efforts with ergogenic aids, and to those sport scientists around the world who have conducted research in order to evaluate the effectiveness of numerous ergogenic aids. Special thanks go to Rainer Martens for the suggestion and encouragement to develop this book, and to Marie Roy, the developmental editor, for her expert guidance and responsiveness throughout all phases of production. Sincere appreciation is extended to John Wentworth, copy editor, and Phaedra Hise, Christine Drews, Steve Otto, and Valerie Hall, assistant editors, for a superb job; also to Dick Flood, the cartoonist, and Admakers, the graphic artists, for their remarkable renditions of my cartoon ideas. Finally, many thanks to Jeanne Kruger for her assistance in preparation of the final copy.

How to Use This Book

THE PURPOSE OF THIS BOOK is to provide an overall review and analysis of the available scientific evidence relative to the effectiveness of a wide variety of special aids to human athletic performance. The focus is on some of the most common ergogenic aids that athletes have tried throughout the years. The book is designed to be a reference source to help the athlete make an informed decision regarding the use of ergogenic aids as a means of improving sports performance.

The book is divided into seven chapters. The first two chapters provide the theoretical background for the use of ergogenic aids by athletes. Chapter 1 gives the reader a broad overview of ergogenic aids in sport. Chapter 2 focuses on human energy, which is the key to athletic performance and the means by which ergogenic aids might help the athlete. The remaining five chapters focus on five general categories of ergogenic aids. Chapter 3 covers nutritional ergogenic aids, such as carbohydrate loading; chapter 4 deals with pharmacological ergogenic aids, such as stimulants and depressants; chapter 5 analyzes the research with physiological ergogenic aids, such as blood doping; chapter 6 focuses on psychological energizers and tranquilizers; and chapter 7 discusses mechanical and biomechanical ergogenic aids, such as sportswear and sports equipment.

In the last five chapters the discussion of each special aid has three parts. First, the theoretical basis for the use of the aid is indicated. (In other words, how the aid is supposed to modify energy utilization in order to improve performance.) Second, a summary of the key scientific research findings is presented. Finally, a general recommendation is offered.

I recommend you read the entire book to obtain a proper perspective of the use of ergogenic aids in sports. However, if you are interested in a specific aid, you may wish to focus your attention on the appropriate chapter. For any ergogenic aid that interests you, you should review the theoretical basis and the analysis of the scientific data, as these are the criteria on which the general recommendation for use is based.

The general recommendation offered will be tempered by medical, legal, and ethical constraints. If a special aid poses a medical risk to the healthy athlete it cannot be recommended, even if it has been found highly effective. In my opinion, any ergogenic aid considered illegal by such sport-governing authorities as the International Olympic Committee, the National Collegiate Athletic Association, or the National Federation of High School Athletic Associations should also be considered unethical by the athlete. Thus, although I recognize my code of ethics is not universally supported by athletes, no banned ergogenic aid will be recommended in this book.

Chapter 1

Improving Sports Performance—Preliminary Considerations

FOR MANY ATHLETES, WINNING is the predominant goal in sports. Although most of us involved in sports may agree with the implications of the statement, "It is not whether you win or lose, but how you play the game," we all know that it is much more fun to win than to lose. The ultimate goal for many athletes is to win, whether it be an Olympic gold medal or an age-group award in a local road race. Winning might also mean meeting a specific, personal performance goal—for the elite athlete, a new world record for the 1,500-meter run; for the local road runner, a personal best of 40 minutes in a 10-kilometer run.

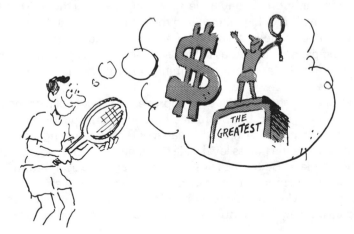

Most athletes train long and hard to achieve their performance goals, and this is the most effective approach. But among some of the questions the athlete, elite or otherwise, faces are, How can I improve my ability to win? How can I break the record? And when the goals of winning and breaking records in sports become valued or perhaps overly valued, some athletes will use any means possible, including illegal ones, to attain them.

Among the means available to the athlete are *ergogenic aids*—special substances, methods, or equipment designed to improve performance. Many of these aids are legal and readily available to you; others are illegal and possibly harmful. The purpose of this book is to provide an overall review and analysis of the available scientific evidence relative to the effectiveness of a wide variety of special aids to human athletic performance. The book is designed to be a reference source to help all those involved in sport make an informed decision regarding the use of ergogenic aids as a means of improving sports performance.

A discussion of the various ergogenic aids and how you may use them follows in chapters 3 through 7. But first let's consider the reason that athletic records continue to be broken and the limits that exist in human performance.

Improvement in Physical Performance

With few exceptions, the constant improvement in physical performance and the resultant breaking of established records in sports has continued unabated for the past 100 years. Not so long ago the 4-minute mile, the 7-foot high jump, and the 15-foot pole vault were considered ultimate performances in sport. Today athletes are approaching the 3:40-mile (see Figure 1.1), the 8-foot high jump, and the 20-foot pole vault. Similar comparisons can be made in a variety of sports at national and international levels of competition, as well as in high schools and colleges. In some sports high school athletes are now performing better than Olympic champions did 30 years ago.

Achievement in sport continues to improve for a variety of reasons. Larger population and greater opportunities for sport participation increase the genetic pool of potential record breakers. Better coaching and training methods improve the fitness level, skill technique, and psychological strategies of the athlete. Better facilities, nutrition, and medical treatment help the athlete to train more effectively. Technological improvements in equipment design provide mechanical or biomechanical advantages. Individually and collectively, these are the major reasons sports records continue to be broken.

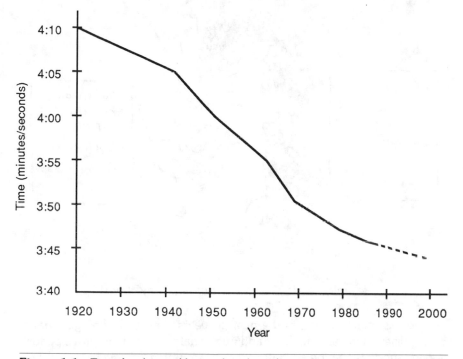

Figure 1.1   Time for the world record in the mile run has decreased since 1920.

Limits to Physical Performance

Are there limits to human physical and athletic performance? If so, what are they? In my mind, the ultimate barrier in performance is the optimal production and utilization of *energy*, for energy is the basis of all movement in sport.

The two primary factors contributing to energy production and utilization in sport are genetic endowment and training. Heredity provides us all with certain physical abilities to produce energy. To succeed in sport we need to maximize or control our ability to produce energy and use it in the most efficient manner possible. Even if we are born with the characteristics of a natural athlete, we have to train hard to realize our potential.

At present, intervention with genetic potential as a means of enhancing sports performance has not been applied extensively (although some concern exists that the advent of genetic engineering may eventually lead to such intervention). On the other hand, the application of science to sport

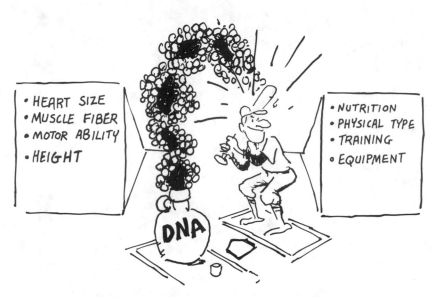

Heredity deals the cards, but you play them.

training has mushroomed in the past 20 years. Sport physiologists have studied different training methods and nutritional practices to improve performance; sport psychologists have utilized a number of psychological approaches to remove mental barriers to performance; motor-learning specialists and biomechanists have investigated optimal means to learn and execute specific sports skills. Much of this research has focused on ways to lower barriers to human performance.

There are three general types of barriers to optimal performance in sports that can be somewhat controlled: physiological, psychological, and biomechanical. *Physiological barriers* limit the ability to produce energy. *Psychological barriers* limit the ability to control energy. *Biomechanical barriers* limit the ability to utilize energy most efficiently. The three barriers may be interrelated. For example, a psychological barrier to performance may interfere with optimal production of energy by physiological processes and may also disrupt optimal biomechanical utilization of energy.

An extended discussion of the production, utilization, and control of energy and associated fatigue processes appears in the next chapter. At this point it will be sufficient to note some of the physiological, psychological, and biomechanical limitations to human performance. Figure 1.2 highlights some of these barriers.

Although you cannot modify your genetic potential (you did not get a chance to choose your parents), you can maximize what you do have through training. You might not have the natural athletic ability of another,

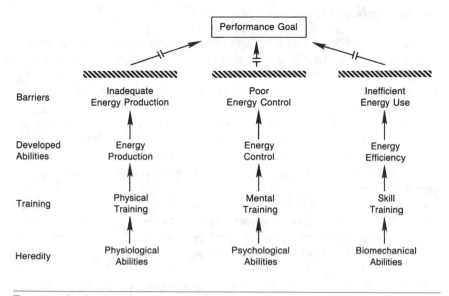

Figure 1.2   Inadequate energy production, poor energy control, and inefficient energy use may be barriers to achieving performance goals.

but proper training can develop your inherited abilities to the level necessary to achieve your goal. As will be emphasized throughout this book, proper training is the most effective way to improve athletic performance.

Ergogenic Aids

Through the means of *ergogenic aids* attempts have been made to improve athletic performance above and beyond that which may occur through natural ability and training. *Ergogenic* is derived from the Greek words *ergon* (work) and *gennan* (to produce). Hence, ergogenic is usually interpreted as work producing or work enhancing. The science of ergonomics has been applied extensively to business and industry to increase work output, ranging from the most effective chair design for increased secretarial comfort and work productivity to the production of complex robots to facilitate automobile assembly. In this sense we all use some form of ergogenic aid in our normal daily tasks to make work easier or to increase productivity. For me, the word processor and the specially designed back chair I am now using to produce this manuscript are two effective ergogenic aids—along with several cups of coffee to stimulate my mental processes at 5:30 in the morning.

Energy Enhancement

In order to be effective as a means of improving performance in sports, ergogenic aids, or *special aids*, must benefit human energy production, energy control, or energy efficiency. All three of these aspects of energy are important to all sports in one way or another, but one of them may be predominant.

Energy production must occur rapidly in order for an athlete to succeed in an event involving power or high speed, such as the 100-meter dash. Conversely, success in endurance events, such as the 26.2 mile marathon, depends on the ability to sustain energy production at an optimal level for hours.

Energy control is important in events where the athlete must respond rapidly to changing stimuli, such as a tennis player reacting to the movement of the ball. Putting in golf is another example of an event in which energy control is critical. Anxiety at this time may disrupt precise energy control, resulting in a missed putt.

Energy efficiency is also critical for success in most sports. For example, much of the recent improvement in swimming records might be attributed to more efficient stroke mechanics, resulting in more propulsive force to pull the swimmer through the water. However, part of the improvement may also be due to a more efficient swimsuit design—particularly for female swimmers—that reduces resistance to movement in water.

In order to be applied to athletics, ergogenic aids must theoretically be able to enhance some process of energy utilization necessary for success in a given sport. For example, caffeine is theorized to enhance performance in prolonged endurance events, such as marathon running, due to its theoretical value to affect neural and hormonal systems and to help preserve optimal energy sources in the muscle for the latter stages of the race. Anabolic steroids are theorized to improve performance in sports involving strength and power due to their alleged ability to increase muscle mass.

The timing of the use of the special aid is also an important consideration. Caffeine is often used within an hour or two of the actual competition, whereas anabolic steroids have been used primarily in conjunction with the training process months prior to the time of competition.

One must also consider the possible detrimental effects of special aids, not only in relation to athletic performance but also to the overall health of the athlete. For example, caffeine ingestion raises heat production in the body (ever notice how warm you get after drinking a cup of coffee?) and acts as a diuretic on the kidneys to increase fluid losses. Both of these effects may hamper the athlete's ability to tolerate exercise in a warm environment, possibly impairing performance. The prolonged use of anabolic steroids has been associated with a wide variety of health problems, ranging from mild cases of acne to serious liver disease.

Types of Ergogenic Aids

Athletes have been using special aids in attempts to improve performance since the early days of civilization and organized sports competition. In ancient Greece and Rome much of the focus was on nutritional aids. For example, athletes may have believed that in specific body organs of animals were located certain attributes, such as the courage of the lion in its heart, which could be transferred to the athletes if they consumed the organs. One report noted that athletes consumed the milk of an Arctic reindeer in heat (for whatever purpose—your guess is as good as mine). Over 100 years ago numerous athletes—including boxers, marathon runners, baseball and soccer players, European cyclists, Olympians, and others— experimented with such drugs as alcohol, caffeine, and cocaine in attempts to improve their athletic abilities. In recent years the phenomenal increase in sports science research has paralleled the development of virtually hundreds of different ergogenic aids aimed at lowering barriers to human athletic performance.

There are a variety of ways to classify ergogenic aids to sports performance, but for the purpose of this book five different categories will be used: *nutritional aids*, *physiological aids*, *psychological aids*, *pharmacological aids*, and *mechanical and biomechanical aids*. It should be noted, however, that this is an arbitrary classification, as an ergogenic aid may exert its effect across several categories. For example, caffeine is technically a drug (pharmacological aid), but is also contained in several foods and beverages we consume (nutritional aid) and may affect a variety of human metabolic processes (physiological aid) and mental processes (psychological aid).

Table 1.1 lists some of the special aids that either have been used or are currently being used by athletes in a wide variety of sports.

Promotion of Ergogenic Aids

Athletes at all levels of competition have gone to extraordinary lengths in their training programs in order to help insure victory against an opponent or to establish a new standard or record of performance. And, to be sure, adequate and proper training is the most effective means of enhancing athletic performance goals.

However, many athletes wonder if there is any special aid that will improve performance above and beyond that attributable to training. They continue to search for substances or techniques that will provide them with an advantage over their competitors—the so-called racer's edge—or with the ability to exceed their own personal best and/or set new records. Communication with elite athletes has revealed that prior to competition they

---

TABLE 1.1
FIVE CLASSES OF ERGOGENIC AIDS

NUTRITIONAL AIDS   **PHYSIOLOGICAL AIDS**

Amino acid supplements   Alkaline salts

Carbohydrate loading   Blood doping

Water   Oxygen

PHARMACOLOGICAL AIDS   **PSYCHOLOGICAL AIDS**

Amphetamines   Hypnosis

Anabolic steroids   Imagery

Caffeine   Stress management

MECHANICAL/BIOMECHANICAL AIDS

Body composition

Clothing

Equipment

---

are in such a frame of mind that they will take anything in order to increase performance, provided it is not actually lethal. Athletes at lower levels of competition exhibit similar attitudes and behaviors; they consume a variety of nutritional compounds in the belief that performance will be enhanced.

As long as athletes believe that a magical compound exists to improve performance, entrepreneurs will continue to market products designed to capitalize on these beliefs. Recent examples of "magical compounds" include bee pollen, vitamin B_{15}, and special amino acid mixtures.

How effective are the various ergogenic aids? Do they reliably improve athletic performance? If you read certain sport magazines you may get the impression that certain nutritional compounds are essential to maximal performance. For example, one leading journal for bodybuilders often contains articles detailing the benefits of protein or amino acid supplements as a means of increasing muscle mass and strength. However, the publisher of this journal happens to market a variety of expensive protein and amino acid supplements and advertises them extensively in this same journal. The author of the article is protected by the first amendment; thus

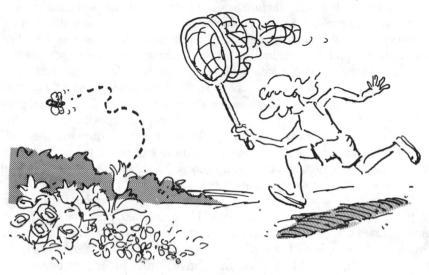

"I need that bee pollen!"

he or she may express the opinion that these supplements may significantly improve performance. On the other hand, advertisements are regulated by the Federal Trade Commission and may not contain any unproven claims. As an astute observer you should be able to understand why the publisher would print the article and the advertisement in proximity to each other. Advertisers may also market their products using star athletes, whose personal testimony about the product's effectiveness may also be covered by the first amendment.

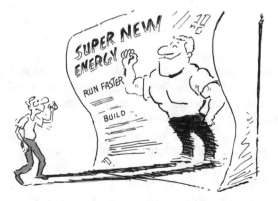

Advertisements in some sports magazines may make some misleading claims.

Companies that manufacture special aids to athletic performance are in business to make a profit. To further this objective, the truth about a product, particularly nutritional aids, might be stretched somewhat. For example, research has shown that distance runners may use slightly greater amounts of their muscle protein while training on a daily basis. Although this protein could be replaced easily by simply consuming a slightly greater amount of protein in the daily diet, one company marketed a special protein mixture for distance runners designed to replace specific amino acids that the runners might use. Although the mixture the company was selling was quality protein, it was also much more expensive than an equivalent amount of high-quality protein that could be obtained from such natural sources as milk or low-fat meat, fish, or poultry.

So how do you know whether or not a particular ergogenic aid will help to improve your performance in sports? Unfortunately, personal testimony, unsupported articles, and deceptive advertisements in certain popular sports journals often serve as the basis for judging the value of a given aid. As already noted, such information may have some underlying biases.

Fortunately, many of the available special aids to sports performance have received considerable attention by various sport scientists, who have made available some research data to evaluate their effectiveness. In general, sport scientists have no inherent interest in the special aid; thus they can provide an unbiased evaluation of the aid's ability to improve performance.

However, as we shall see throughout this book, not all research is in agreement regarding the effectiveness of some ergogenic aids. In many cases the disparity may be due to differences in the designs of the studies, for some of the older studies with ergogenic aids did not control outside factors that may have influenced the results of the study.

Placebo Effect

One factor that can influence a study's findings is the placebo effect. A *placebo* is an inactive substance. Placebos are often utilized in medicine for patients who demand a prescription yet have no physical disease that necessitates medication. Physicians recognize that many illnesses are psychosomatic in nature, so a harmless placebo drug is prescribed. Placebos possess potentially powerful psychological effects. Often these agents are effective in curing the patient's problem, resulting in what is known as the *placebo effect*.

The placebo effect may occur in sports as well. I recall the trainer of my high school football team would give us dextrose pills before each game and suggest they would provide us with extra energy. Although today I realize these pills were nothing but sugar, at the time I thought they would

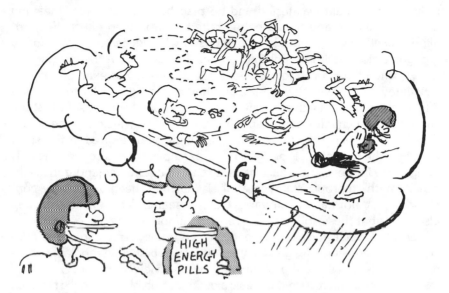

Believing in "magic" of a pill may produce a placebo effect.

provide us with an advantage over our opponents. However, our final record was 3 wins, 6 losses, and a tie, so the pills apparently were not effective either as an authentic ergogenic aid or as a placebo.

If you read about an ergogenic aid that appears to be safe, buy it, try it, and find that it appears to make you feel better in training or competition, you may be experiencing the placebo effect. The aid may work for you not because of any bona fide physiological or mechanical advantage it provides but simply because you believe in it, which may benefit you psychologically. Although the use of the placebo effect may have some application to sports under certain circumstances, it must be eliminated in well-controlled research with ergogenic aids.

Research Considerations

We do not want to spend a lot of time discussing how to design the perfect study to evaluate the effectiveness of various ergogenic aids, but the placebo effect is a very important consideration not only for research purposes but also for your own understanding of how certain special aids may work for athletes. Throughout this book I will be noting that some studies suffer from improper methodology or experimental design, thus limiting the interpretation of their results. This may mean several things. First, it could be that only the special aid was tested and no placebo trial was used, meaning positive results, if any, could be attributed to a placebo effect. Second, *blind procedures* might not have been used when necessary: With many ergogenic aids it is important that neither the subject nor the investigator knows when the aid or the placebo is administered. For example, if subjects know they have received the aid they may work harder to prove its effectiveness. An individual not involved in the actual conduct of the study should keep such information and reveal it at the conclusion of the study. Third, the subjects might not have been individuals trained in the sport for which the special aid is designed. For example, studies concerning aids designed to improve endurance capacity should use trained endurance athletes. Fourth, improper statistical analysis may have been used so the conclusions may not have been valid. Other research design problems may also exist, but these four are the most common.

Recent research studies with ergogenic aids usually adhere to sound principles of experimental design. They are usually published in reputable scientific journals in which the study has been reviewed by several other researchers with interests in ergogenic aids. Such published scientific research is the best data available on the effectiveness of various ergogenic aids. Still, it should be noted that the results of a single research study do not prove or disprove the value of a given ergogenic aid—although certain entrepreneurs would like us to believe otherwise. Several years ago advertisements started to appear in runners' magazines extolling the virtues of fructose (a simple sugar) as the best means of providing carbohydrate energy sources during long-distance running. The results of a single study were used as the basis for the advertising claims. Later research did not support these initial findings. Thus, the value of special aids to athletic performance should be supported by a number of well-controlled research studies.

It should also be noted that the results reported in scientific journals usually focus upon the effect of an ergogenic aid on a group of individuals. However, although all humans share similar anatomical and physiological traits, we all possess biological individuality due to either basic hereditary differences or environmental modifications. For example, the response you may have to caffeine prior to a competitive event may depend on whether or not you are a habitual user of caffeine. Although caffeine is theorized to improve performance, it may actually be detrimental to some individuals who do not normally consume caffeine.

In later chapters you will be given recommendations and guidelines regarding the use of some specific ergogenic aids. However, I believe it is important for you to get the big picture as to why various ergogenic aids are used. Thus, the next chapter will focus upon energy and fatigue processes in sport, which will help to serve as a basis for understanding the specific applications of ergogenic aids to enhance performance in a wide variety of sports.

Selected Readings

If you would like to read more detailed accounts of the various ergogenic aids, particularly more of the scientific details, the following sources should be very helpful, as they served as the scientific basis for this chapter. A list such as this one follows each chapter. Basically, only two general sources are listed, books and reviews. Books provide broad coverage of specific topics, whereas reviews provide a contemporary synthesis of the experimental research. In some cases, particularly when an ergogenic aid is relatively new and insufficient research is available to develop a review, specific research studies may be listed.

Books

Landers, D. (Ed.). (1986). *Sport and elite performers.* Champaign, IL: Human Kinetics.

Morgan, W. (Ed.). (1972). *Ergogenic aids and muscular performance.* New York: Academic Press.

Williams, M. (Ed.). (1983). *Ergogenic aids in sport.* Champaign, IL: Human Kinetics.

Reviews

Clarke, D., & Eckert, H. (Eds.). (1985). Limits of human performance. *American Academy of Physical Education Papers,* **18**, 1-137.

Coyle, E. (1984). Ergogenic aids. *Clinics in Sports Medicine,* **3**, 731-742.

Percy, E. (1977). Athletic aids: Fact or fiction. *Canadian Medical Association Journal,* **117**, 601-645.

Chapter 2

Energy and
Sports Performance

ENERGY EXISTS IN A VARIETY of forms in nature. Light energy is emitted from the sun. Electrical energy is produced during lightning storms. Nuclear energy is generated from fissionable materials. Chemical energy is stored in food and other materials. Heat energy is released in the body, which helps to maintain our temperature at 98.6 degrees Fahrenheit. Mechanical energy is movement.

A key principle involving energy is that *one form of energy may be converted into another*. For example, in a nuclear power plant uranium may be the source of nuclear energy to produce heat energy; the heat energy may be used to generate mechanical energy by producing steam to move a turbine; the movement of the turbine may generate electrical energy, which may eventually reach a lamp in our house for the release of light energy. Through the process of civilization scientists have learned to control much of the energy in nature to help make our lives easier and more comfortable.

Sport scientists have also been investigating the optimal application of energy principles to human physical performance. For our purposes, the two principal forms of energy important to sport are *chemical energy* and *mechanical energy*. Chemical energy is stored in our bodies in a variety of forms and is used to produce mechanical energy, which results in movement.

Two other forms of energy produced in the body may also affect sports performance. *Heat energy* is generated continuously in our bodies, but may increase markedly during exercise. Excess production or losses of body heat during exercise may impair optimal performance. *Electrochemical energy* produced by our nervous system is necessary for our muscles to contract and produce movement. Just as a telephone system uses electricity to allow us to communicate with each other, the nervous system uses electricity, in the form of ions, to allow our brain to communicate with our muscles. Any disruption in the production or proper application of this electrochemical energy in the body may lead to suboptimal performance.

As in the previous example of the nuclear power plant, your body can also change energy from one form to another. For example, the chemical energy found in a glass of orange juice could be converted into an equivalent amount of a different form of chemical energy and stored in the body. This chemical energy, if totally converted to other forms of energy, would provide the average adult male with enough mechanical energy to climb 2,000 feet, create enough heat energy to raise his body temperature 3 degrees Fahrenheit, or provide him with the electrical energy equivalent of 7,000 watts.

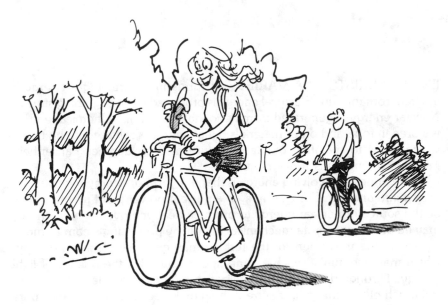

Optimal sports performance depends on optimal energy, and basically there are three principles involved: type, utilization, and control of energy. These principles will be elaborated on in the sections that follow: human energy systems and fuels (principles of type and utilization) and human energy control and efficiency (principle of control). For now, though, let's illustrate these principles by use of an analogy that may be drawn between your body and an automobile.

First, *you must have enough of the right type of chemical energy*, or fuel, stored in your body. Most cars function properly on ordinary gasoline, some need premium grades, and high-speed competition race cars demand special mixtures for optimal performance. Like a car, your body runs on fuel. The type of fuel your body uses depends on the energy demands of a given sport. As you shall see, your muscles store several different types of chemical energy, or fuel, some of which are designed for high-power output and others for endurance.

Second, *you must be able to utilize your chemical energy sources* at an optimal rate. Putting a special fuel mixture in the family station wagon will not convert it into an Indy 500 competitor, for the family car does not have the engine capable of using the special fuel at a fast enough rate. To extend the analogy, your muscles are your engines. They must be capable of processing your chemical-energy sources at a rate optimal for specific sports. For some sports you need powerful engines to produce energy rapidly for short periods of time; in other sports you need smaller, more efficient engines to produce energy for prolonged periods.

Third, *you must be able to control energy* so that you are efficient in meeting the mechanical demands of the sport. For a racing car this may mean a design that maximizes the application of energy to forward propulsion, such as special gears and tires, and minimizes negative energy forces, such as the reduction in wind resistance through proper streamlining techniques and drafting. Although movement efficiency is an important consideration in all sports, an appropriate comparison here is the sport of swimming. The swimmer must learn the most effective technique of producing propulsive forces for movement through the water, such as the proper position of the arm and hand during the pull phase, while at the same time reducing negative forces by modifying body position or using special swimsuits to create a streamlined effect.

In order to understand the application of ergogenic aids as a means of improving sports performance, you need to understand how the human body stores and utilizes energy and about the possible causes of impairment, such as fatigue or inefficient utilization.

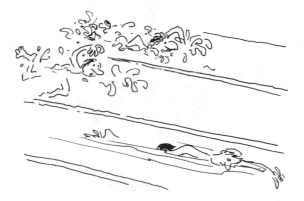

Success often depends on <u>controlling</u> energy, not just expending it!

Energy Systems and Fuels

As you remember from chapter 1, energy production must occur rapidly in order to be successful in high-power or high-speed athletic events. In contrast, success in endurance events depends on the ability to sustain energy production at an optimal level for hours. For these different activities, different energy systems and fuels are used in the muscle.

Muscle Fiber Types

Muscles provide the means for human movement by contracting (shortening) and moving the bones to which they are attached. Figure 2.1 provides an illustration of a muscle connecting to a bone via its tendon. Each whole muscle contains varying numbers of *motor units*, and each motor unit is composed of varying numbers of individual *muscle cells* or *fibers*. One of the key points for our discussion is that muscle fibers come in different types (although all fibers in each individual motor unit are of the same type), based primarily on the speed at which they contract. A single contraction of a fiber is known as a *twitch*. In general, some muscle fibers shorten at a fast rate of speed and are known as *fast-twitch* (FT) muscle fibers, whereas others shorten at a slower rate and are known as *slow-twitch* (ST) muscle fibers.

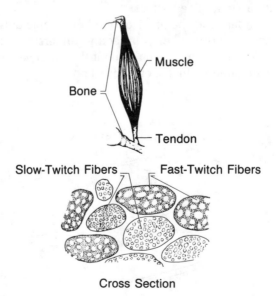

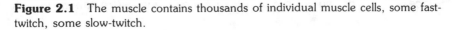

Figure 2.1 The muscle contains thousands of individual muscle cells, some fast-twitch, some slow-twitch.

Energy Systems and ATP

The rate of speed at which a muscle fiber contracts depends on its ability to convert its chemical energy into mechanical energy, the latter being the actual shortening of the muscle cell. Your muscles contain three distinct systems that determine the rate of energy production for movement. One is the *ATP-CP system*, the second is the *lactic acid system*, and the third is the *oxygen system*. Although each muscle fiber possesses all three energy systems, the dominance of one system over another will determine the energy characteristics of the individual muscle fiber.

Although your muscles possess three different energy systems, only one form of energy can be utilized to cause the muscle to contract. This form is *ATP*, the abbreviation for *adenosine triphosphate*, a high-energy chemical compound natural in all muscle cells. When your muscle is stimulated by a nerve impulse, a series of events occurs, leading to the breakdown of ATP, the release of chemical energy, and the harnessing of this energy for muscle contraction (see Figure 2.2). ATP is the immediate and essential source of energy for muscle contraction. Without it, your muscle cannot contract. However, the muscle contains only a small amount of ATP, about enough for you to expend energy at your maximal rate for only one second. If muscle contraction is to continue, additional ATP must be supplied. The faster you want your muscles to contract, the more rapidly you must replenish ATP. The purpose of the three energy systems is to supply this additional ATP, but the rate at which they can supply it varies.

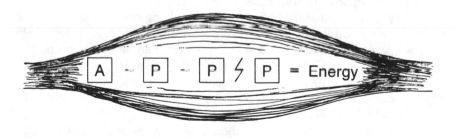

Figure 2.2 Adenosine triphosphate (ATP) is the immediate source of energy for muscle contraction. When the end phosphate is split off, energy is released.

ATP-CP System. The ATP-CP energy system consists of *ATP* and *CP* (*creatine phosphate*), another high-energy phosphate compound. ATP is the immediate source of energy for muscle contraction. It may release energy very rapidly, but it is in very limited supply. CP may also break down and release energy very rapidly, but this energy cannot be used directly for muscle contraction. Instead it is used to rapidly resynthesize ATP (see Figure 2.3). However, CP supply is also limited in the muscle and may only be able to resynthesize ATP for an additional 4 to 5 seconds. The ability to use ATP and CP rapidly is a primary characteristic of the FT muscle fibers. It is interesting that this energy system does not need oxygen (aerobic) in order to perform and thus is an *anaerobic* (without oxygen) source of energy. The ATP-CP energy system is capable of producing energy rapidly for short periods of time.

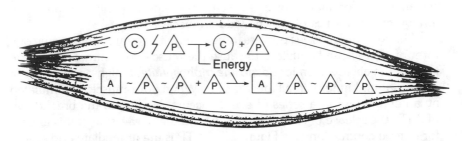

Figure 2.3   Creatine phosphate splits to release energy for the rapid resynthesis of ATP.

Lactic Acid System.   The lactic acid energy system uses carbohydrates as fuel, primarily in the form of glycogen stored in the muscles. The breakdown of *muscle glycogen* is known as *glycogenolysis*. It leads to a process called *glycolysis*, in which ATP can be produced rapidly, although not as rapidly as compared to the breakdown of CP.

Glycolysis may occur both in the presence and absence of oxygen. Under normal resting conditions the need of your muscles for ATP is relatively low, so glycolysis proceeds at a slower rate and can be sustained by the oxygen you take in. This aerobic energy production from carbohydrate accounts for about 40 percent of your energy demands at rest. As you begin to exercise, the rate of *aerobic glycolysis* increases to help meet your need for additional ATP.

However, glycolysis that occurs without oxygen also contributes to energy production. As you pick up your speed, you will eventually reach a point where aerobic glycolysis is inadequate to support energy production. Proportionally more of the ATP is now produced without adequate oxygen, through *anaerobic glycolysis* (see Figure 2.4). Through a series of chemical reactions in the muscle cell, the formation of lactic acid allows anaerobic glycolysis to continue. Unfortunately, the accumulation of *excess* lactic acid has been associated with fatigue processes within the muscle cell, so there is a limit to this energy system during exercise. Thus, the lactic acid energy system is capable of producing energy at a fairly rapid rate, but it alone cannot produce energy for prolonged periods.

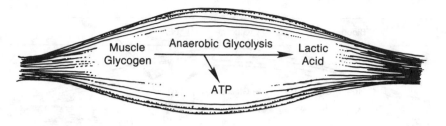

Figure 2.4 In the lactic acid energy system, muscle glycogen (carbohydrate) can break down to form ATP in the absence of adequate oxygen, but lactic acid is formed.

Oxygen System. The oxygen energy system can use a variety of fuels to produce ATP, but depends primarily on *carbohydrates* and *fats*. The main source of carbohydrate for muscular energy during exercise is glucose, which, as noted before, is stored in limited supplies in the muscle as glycogen. Additional glucose is stored in the liver as glycogen and may be released into the blood for delivery to the muscle when needed, although the supply in the liver is also limited. The main source of fat for muscular energy during exercise is *free fatty acids* (FFA). Some *fats*, known as *triglycerides*, are stored in limited supply in the muscle and may break down into FFA for entry into the oxygen energy system. However, much of the fat in our body is stored just under the skin and in some deeper areas, and these sources can provide substantial amounts of FFA. Normally, *protein* is not used for energy production to any great extent, but under some conditions protein may become a significant source of energy for the oxygen energy system.

As its name implies, the oxygen energy system needs an adequate supply of oxygen delivered to the muscles to help release the chemical energy stored in carbohydrates and fats. In contrast to the two anaerobic energy systems, the oxygen energy system is *aerobic* in nature. Figure 2.5 provides a graphic overview of the oxygen energy system and its fuel sources.

Although the oxygen system cannot produce ATP as rapidly as the two anaerobic systems, it is capable of producing greater quantities of ATP at a somewhat slower rate. Moreover, the rate at which the oxygen energy system may produce ATP depends on the type of fuel. For a given amount of oxygen, you may produce more work if you use carbohydrate instead of fat. In other words, carbohydrate is a more efficient fuel than fat. Unfortunately, the ability to store carbohydrate in the body is limited for certain prolonged endurance events, whereas the body's fat supplies are rather extensive. Thus, while the oxygen energy system is designed for endurance, the availability of the optimal fuel may limit performance.

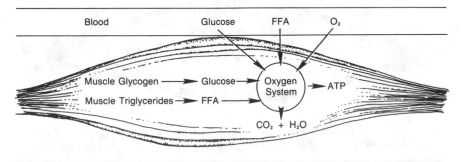

Figure 2.5   The oxygen system uses mostly carbohydrates and fats stored in the muscle or delivered by the blood as fuels.

Rates of Energy Production and Fiber Type

As noted previously, there are several different muscle fiber types in the body, and for our purposes we have classified them as fast-twitch (FT) and slow-twitch (ST) fibers. Both types of muscle fibers need to use ATP as the immediate source of energy for muscle contraction, but the rate at which they are able to replenish ATP is different. Both muscle fiber types are able to use all three human energy systems to produce energy, but the FT muscle fibers will use primarily the ATP-CP and lactic acid energy systems, whereas the ST fibers will use primarily the oxygen system. As noted, the oxygen system cannot replenish ATP as rapidly as the other two systems.

The different muscle fiber types you possess appear to be related to the success in specific types of sports or athletic endeavors. Let us look briefly at the rates of energy production and their relationship to sports performance, using several events in elite male track athletes as a basis for comparison. In some events, such as the 100-meter dash, athletes need to produce energy very rapidly for a very short period of time, say 10 seconds or so. In this case, a high percentage of the energy is derived from the ATP-CP system, so individuals with greater proportions of FT muscle fibers and highly developed ATP-CP systems may have the greater potential for success. In a 400-meter dash (.25 mile), energy needs to be generated rapidly for a longer period of time, about 45 seconds. In such an event the lactic acid energy system will provide the majority of the energy, so athletes with high capacities for anaerobic glycolysis may be more successful. In longer distances, such as 10,000 meters (6.2 miles), run in about 28 minutes, energy is provided primarily by the oxygen energy system. Thus, individuals with high aerobic capacities are more likely to be successful. Table 2.1 summarizes the characteristics of each of the three energy systems found in the muscle cells.

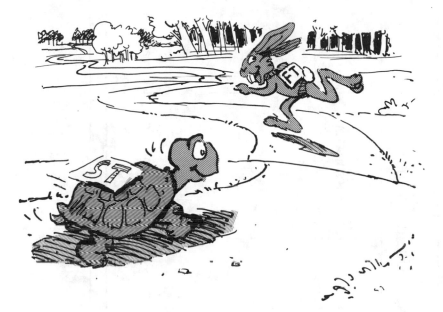

The currently available scientific evidence suggests that each of us is born with our own specific distribution of muscle fiber types—that is, some of us may have a greater proportion of ST muscle fibers and others may have more FT ones. In general, the distribution of muscle fiber types in men and women is similar, and untrained individuals possess about 50 percent of each type, although there is a wide range of distribution. However, research has shown that elite sprinters have a greater proportion of FT fibers and elite distance runners have more ST fibers. It is currently unknown whether the success of these elite athletes is primarily due to the inheritance of the right type of muscle fibers or to the effect that years of training may have as a means of increasing the number of either FT or ST fiber types, but the former appears to be a more plausible explanation for performance at the elite level.

Thus, the amount of each type of muscle fiber you possess may have some important implications for sport. However, although you may not have inherited the potential to perform at the elite level, you may maximize the capacity of each of your three energy systems by proper training. For example, a properly balanced training program for a distance runner will improve the ability of both fiber types to use the oxygen energy system, thus improving the ability to produce energy more rapidly without fatigue over long distances.

TABLE 2.1
MAJOR CHARACTERISTICS OF MUSCLE ENERGY SYSTEMS

	ATP-CP	LACTIC ACID	OXYGEN (CARBOHYDRATE)	OXYGEN (FAT)
Main energy source	ATP, CP	Muscle glycogen	Muscle glycogen	Muscle fats
Exercise intensity	Highest	High	Lower	Lowest
Rate of ATP production	Highest	High	Lower	Lowest
Power production	Highest	High	Lower	Lowest
Capacity for total ATP production	Lowest	Low	High	Highest
Endurance capacity	Lowest	Low	High	Highest
Oxygen needed	No	No	Yes	Yes
Anaerobic/aerobic	Anaerobic	Anaerobic	Aerobic	Aerobic
Characteristic track event	100-meter dash	800-meter run	5- to 42-kilometer run	Ultramarathon
Time factor at maximal use	1 to 10 seconds	30 to 120 seconds	More than 5 minutes	Hours

Supply and Support of the Energy Systems

Although the ability of the three energy systems to produce energy for movement resides in the muscle cell itself, each needs a proper supply and support system in order to function at optimal capacity.

The ATP-CP system, as noted previously, uses ATP as the immediate source of energy for muscular contraction, and all three systems are designed to replace ATP. Thus, CP needs to be replenished in order for this energy system to operate. Actually, the energy released from the breakdown of ATP is used to resynthesize CP. However, the ATP used to resynthesize CP is ultimately derived from the oxygen energy system. This process occurs during the recovery period between contractions.

The lactic acid energy system operates primarily in the FT muscle fibers and uses muscle glycogen, or carbohydrate, as its source of energy. Thus, carbohydrate must be replenished in the FT fibers in order for this energy system to function adequately. Moreover, the accumulation of lactic acid in the muscle cell has been indentified as a factor in the development of fatigue, so it must be removed rapidly.

The oxygen energy system operates primarily in the ST muscle fibers. To function properly, it needs an adequate supply of oxygen as well as replenishment of the proper fuel, either muscle glycogen or free fatty acids (FFA).

Moreover, each of the three energy systems needs an adequate supply of various vitamins and minerals in order to function effectively. For example, the B vitamins are essential for processing carbohydrate and fat as energy sources in the muscle cell, whereas calcium, magnesium, sodium, potassium, and iron are critical for regulating various physiological processes within the cell. Also, as one of the byproducts of energy production for movement in the body is heat, the body must be able to dissipate this excess heat in order to function at an optimal level. In this regard, water is one of the most essential nutrients to athletes when exercising under warm or hot environmental conditions.

The *cardiovascular system*, consisting of the heart and blood vessels, is the primary support system because it transports blood to and from the muscle cell. As blood flows through the body it picks up oxygen from the respiratory system in the lungs; glucose from the liver; FFA from the fat (adipose) tissue; a wide variety of nutrients, including vitamins and minerals, and water from the digestive system; and hormones, such as *adrenalin*, from the endocrine system for delivery to the muscle cells in support of energy production. The blood also removes byproducts of energy metabolism, such as lactic acid and excess heat, that can interfere with optimal energy production within the muscle cell (see Figure 2.6).

Thus, in order to perform in sport at an optimal level, an individual must have not only proper development of the appropriate energy system within the muscle cells, but also well-developed supply and support systems. Improvement in the supply and support systems may lead to improved energy production within the muscle cells.

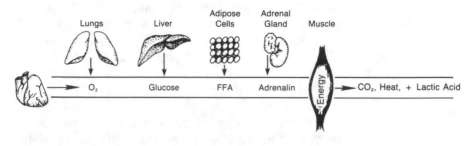

Figure 2.6   The blood is the main supply system to the muscles during exercise as it picks up and delivers oxygen, nutrients, and hormones from other tissues and removes byproducts of energy metabolism.

Energy Control and Efficiency

To optimize your performance in sports, you need to be able to produce and use your energy in the most efficient manner specific to a given sport. You do this primarily through proper training, which enables your nervous system to do two things: to call into play the proper muscle groups, and to control the rate at which energy is expended in those muscles. One of the basic principles of training is *specificity*, of which there are two types: *neuromuscular specificity* (use of proper muscle groups) and *metabolic specificity* (rate of energy expenditure).

The Nervous System and Control of Muscle Function

You are probably aware that the nervous system controls most of your body's functions, including movement. It does so by creating electrical impulses that are transmitted over nerve cells, called *neurons*. Neural stimulation of a particular body tissue initiates a response that is characteristic of that tissue. For example, neural stimulation of your adrenal gland may lead to a release of adrenalin into your blood, whereas stimulation of your muscle cell will cause it to contract and cause movement.

Figure 2.7 represents a simplified schematic of a *neural pathway* between the brain and a muscle cell. An electrical impulse may be generated by a specific neuron in an area of the brain that controls the muscles. This impulse then passes along the neuron down to your spinal cord, where it communicates with another neuron. An electrical impulse is generated in this neuron, which in turn communicates with specific muscle fibers within a large muscle and initiates a muscle contraction.

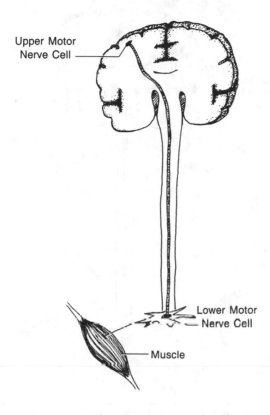

Upper Motor
Nerve Cell

Lower Motor
Nerve Cell

Muscle

Figure 2.7 Voluntary movement is initiated in the motor control center in the brain. The simple pathway illustrated here represents a direct pathway between the brain and the motor nerve cell in the spinal cord.

Unfortunately, the control of human movement, particularly the complex movement patterns found in most sports, is not that simple. The central nervous system, including numerous parts of the brain and the spinal cord, functions as a rapidly acting computer. It receives input, analyzes this input, and then generates output.

During most sports the *central nervous system* receives a wide variety of information (input) from various receptors in our body, including our eyes, inner ears, muscles, and joints. The central nervous system processes this information rapidly and initiates impulses to the necessary muscles for the desired movement patterns (output). Figure 2.8 illustrates some of the neural control mechanisms for human movement (but be aware that this illustration is a gross oversimplification).

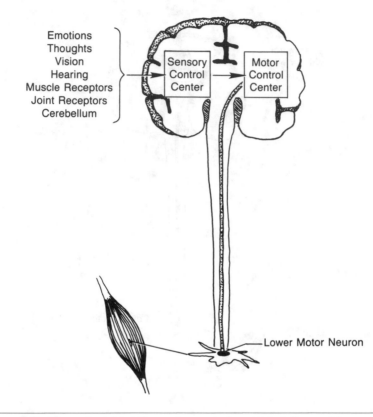

Figure 2.8   The output from the motor control center is influenced by various sensory control centers in different parts of the brain.

Think about the first time you tried a complex sport skill, such as serving a tennis ball, swimming the front crawl, or skiing parallel turns. Do you remember how hard you would concentrate in order to do the skill properly? However, as you practiced repeatedly, the skill became almost second nature and needed less concentration. One theory of learning suggests that as you learn to perform a complex sport skill your central nervous system develops a kind of computerized program for that skill and that a given stimulus will trigger a set pattern of muscular responses. For example, after having perfected your tennis serve, simply throwing the ball into the air may initiate a programmed sequence in your nervous system that eventually results in the proper sequence and timing of muscle contractions and a smooth movement pattern.

For optimal efficiency in sports it is critical to learn and perfect the most effective techniques or skills that enhance success. Another goal when training athletes in complex sport skills may be to get to the point where the skill becomes second nature, so that the athlete can concentrate on other aspects of the competition.

We can see that the nervous system plays an essential role as the control center for human movement. By learning to perform a sport skill efficiently through proper coaching and much practice, your nervous system develops a programmed sequence of muscular contractions that allows you to perform the skill at maximal efficiency and effectiveness, thus spending your energy most productively during competition. This process is often referred to as *neuromuscular specificity of training*, for we train the specific muscles to be used in a given sport. In other words, the best way to become more efficient in bicycling is to use those muscles involved in cycling. Of course cycling muscles are developed best through bicycling, not through swimming or running.

The Nervous System and the Control of Energy

The nervous system not only controls the specific muscles activated to do a particular sport skill, but also controls the amount of energy released in these muscles and how fast this energy is released. In essence, the nerve cells you have in your central nervous system serve specific muscle cells. Some go to the FT muscle fibers; others go to the ST fibers. Of course, as noted above, activation of these fibers will cause either a fast or slow muscle contraction. However, the nervous system controls, in several other ways, the total amount of energy developed. It may activate more muscle fibers, and/or it may activate them more frequently. For example, a nerve fiber that goes to 50 slow-twitch muscle fibers and fires at a rate of 10 impulses per second will not generate nearly as much force as a nerve fiber going to 200 muscle fibers and firing at a rate of 50 per second. As it is the nervous system that control this process, the muscles, in essence, are the slaves of the nervous system.

The nervous system is also important for the control of energy production in that it helps to control the supply and support system to the muscle cells. For example, the nervous system may help to channel the delivery of more blood to the active muscles during exercise, such as to your thigh muscles during bicycling, by opening the blood vessels to those muscles. The nervous system may also stimulate certain glands in the body to secrete hormones in the blood, which may then facilitate fuel supply to and energy production in the muscle cells. One key hormone we shall discuss later is adrenalin, for athletes have taken compounds similar to adrenalin in attempts to improve performance.

In essence, the nervous system controls the three energy systems within the muscle cells. To improve your ability, you have to train the specific energy system or systems needed for a given sport. This process is often referred to as *metabolic specificity of training*. In other words, you need to train at an intensity level comparable to that experienced in competition. If you are training for a 400-meter dash in track, you have to train occasionally at speeds that will stress the lactic acid energy system. You need to train your nervous system to activate your FT fibers more effectively, for they use the lactic acid energy system. As you continue to train, your body will make specific beneficial adjustments in the energy systems within the muscle cells and in the energy support systems, leading to an increased ability to produce energy during exercise.

Controlling the Controller

It is important to realize that the nervous system, as the controller of human movement, needs to function properly in order to achieve optimal performance. Any disturbance in its functioning, such as excessive anxiety, could result in suboptimal performance. Take walking, for example. Walking is a complex motor skill learned early in life. You may not think that walking is a complex skill, but just notice how difficult it is for children to learn to walk properly and develop an efficient style. They stagger all over the place for a while, but eventually learn to become quite efficient. Most of the time you do not have to think about walking. It is a natural skill for you. However, if for some reason you stop and think about walking, such as trying to be extra cool while walking across a stage to pick up an award before hundreds of spectators, the natural skill can become clumsy, and you nearly stumble over your own two feet.

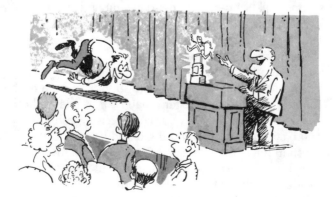

As we shall see throughout this book, a large number and variety of ergogenic aids have been used in efforts to modify nervous system functioning in attempts to improve sports performance. The aids are designed to control the controller in a variety of ways, such as stimulating the nervous system to increase the rate of energy production, decreasing the conscious perception of fatigue, or eliminating the adverse effects of negative thoughts.

Fatigue

The enemy of almost all athletes is fatigue, for the premature development of fatigue will lead to a decrease in athletic performance. Fatigue is a complex phenomenon; it may exist in a variety of forms and have a number of different definitions. For purposes of this book we may define *fatigue* as the inability to utilize your human energy resources to their fullest potential.

The causes of fatigue may be physiological or physical in nature, such as an inadequate energy supply in the muscles, an inability to produce energy rapidly enough, or even an inefficient body composition consisting of too much body fat. Fatigue may also be psychological or mental in nature, such as the inability to concentrate on the task at hand or the improper execution of a sport skill due to mental interference from overstimulation.

Figure 2.9 represents some of the possible *sites of fatigue* in the human body. The following discussion is keyed to the numbers in the figure.

1. One fatigue site may be the motor nerve cells in the brain. Mental tiredness, lack of proper nutrition, and inadequate stimulation or inhibition from other parts of the brain may limit the ability to activate these motor neurons to their optimal potential.
2. The motor nerve cell in the spinal cord leads directly to the muscle. This nerve cell may be inhibited by nerve centers in the brain, by various forms of feedback from the muscles, and by poor nutrition, thus leading to decreased work output.
3. The junction of the nerve ending with the muscle cell may be a fatigue site if inadequate amounts of chemicals are secreted by the nerve ending or if the receptor on the muscle cell does not function properly. In such situations, an electrical impulse would not be generated in the muscle cell to initiate the contraction process.
4. Another source of fatigue could be the inability of the electrical impulse to initiate the contraction process in the muscle. For example, an excess acidity in the muscle cell due to lactic acid accumulation has been theorized to block some of the key steps in the processes that initiate muscle contraction.

5. The muscle cell may also contain inadequate amounts of energy stores, such as carbohydrate in the form of glycogen. Muscle glycogen is the essential fuel source for the lactic acid energy system and is also the most efficient fuel for the oxygen energy system.

6. The blood supply to the muscle is usually not identified as a fatigue site, but for our purposes in discussing ergogenic aids it may be identified as a significant contributing factor to the development of fatigue in the muscle. An inadequate delivery of such nutrients as glucose and FFA, low oxygen levels, and impaired ability to remove lactic acid or heat may adversely affect the performance of both the nervous and muscular systems during exercise.

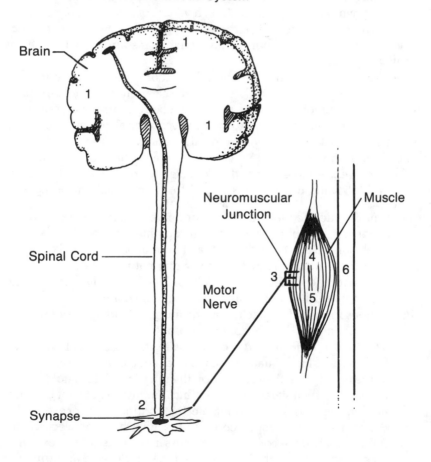

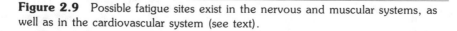

Figure 2.9 Possible fatigue sites exist in the nervous and muscular systems, as well as in the cardiovascular system (see text).

A number of external factors may contribute to the development of fatigue during exercise. In particular, many environmental conditions exert a negative influence on some types of athletic endeavors. For example, endurance performance at altitudes above one mile, such as Denver or Mexico City, will suffer due to the decreased amount of oxygen in the air. High temperatures, wind, and air pollution are other environmental factors that may affect athletic performance.

Another external factor that may influence performance is equipment. One example is the weight of the equipment. All other things equal, using a lightweight racing shoe compared to a heavier training shoe will enable a marathoner to save several minutes covering the standard 26.2 miles.

External factors may increase the physiological energy cost and/or the psychological stress associated with the exercise task and lead to premature development of fatigue.

Ergogenic Aids in Sport: Energy and Fatigue

As previously mentioned, effective training is the most potent ergogenic aid the athlete can use to improve sports performance, primarily by improving energy production, energy processes, and energy efficiency, thereby decreasing fatigue. But, athletes may seek methods that substitute for or augment training; in such cases they turn to ergogenic aids.

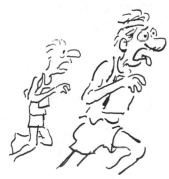
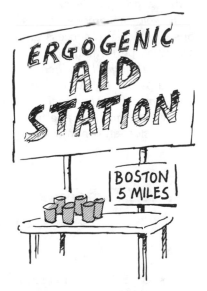

The purpose of most ergogenic aids is to improve sports performance by optimizing energy production and efficiency and thus preventing or delaying the onset of physiological or psychological fatigue. In this regard, various ergogenic aids have been used for the following purposes:

1. To increase psychological processes that maximize energy production
2. To decrease factors that interfere with optimal psychological functioning
3. To increase the amount of muscle tissue in order to generate greater quantities of energy
4. To increase the rate of energy production within the muscle
5. To increase the energy supply in the muscle for greater duration
6. To improve the delivery of energy supplies to the muscle
7. To counteract the accumulation of substances in the body that interfere with optimal energy production
8. To improve the efficiency of human movement

In the following five chapters we shall see how some ergogenic aids have been used successfully, and some unsuccessfully, in attempts to improve athletic performance by optimizing energy utilization and delaying the onset of fatigue.

Nutritional ergogenic aids have been utilized primarily to increase muscle tissue, increase muscle energy supplies, and increase the rate of energy production in the muscle.

Physiological ergogenic aids have been used primarily to increase the rate of energy production in the muscle and to counteract the accumulation of fatigue products.

Psychological ergogenic aids have been used to improve mental conditions conducive to success and to help reduce those mental factors that can impair performance.

Pharmacological ergogenic aids have been utilized for both physiological and psychological reasons.

Mechanical and biomechanical ergogenic aids are designed primarily to improve the mechanical efficiency of human movement, possibly saving both physical and mental energy.

Selected Readings

Books

Brooks, G., & Fahey, T. (1987). *Fundamentals of human performance.* New York: Macmillan.

Jones, N., McCartney, N., & McComas, A. (Eds.). (1986). *Human muscle power*. Champaign, IL: Human Kinetics.

MacDougell, J., Wenger, H., & Green, H. (1982). *Physiological testing of the elite athlete*. Canada: Mutual Press.

McArdle, W., Katch, F., & Katch, V. (1986). *Exercise physiology*. Philadelphia: Lea and Febiger.

Reviews

Gibson, H., & Edwards, R. (1985). Muscular exercise and fatigue. *Sports Medicine, 2*, 120-132.

diPrampero, R. (1981). Energetics of muscular exercise. *Reviews of Physiological and Biochemical Pharmacology, 89*, 143-222.

Williams, M. (1985). Human energy. In M. Williams (Ed.), *Nutritional aspects of human physical and athletic performance* (pp. 20-57). Springfield, IL: Charles C. Thomas.

Chapter 3

Nutritional
Ergogenic Aids

SEVERAL YEARS AGO ROD DIXON and Geoff Smith were involved in one of the most exciting finishes in the New York City Marathon. Smith surged to the lead at about the 15-mile mark while Dixon settled into second place. For the remainder of the race Dixon kept grabbing his hamstring muscles and indicating they were cramping. Smith looked like a sure winner. But as they entered Central Park, Dixon began to close the gap between them. Smith looked like a runner who wants his legs to go faster, but they just would not turn over. Meanwhile Dixon was chipping away at the lead. In the end, Dixon passed Smith. A classic photo of the finish shows Dixon with his arms raised in victory and Smith sprawled on the ground across the finish line. When I watched this dramatic finish on television I wondered if nutrition may have played a role in the outcome.

As noted previously, energy is life. The food you eat provides you with over 50 nutrients essential to life; you would be amazed at the wide variety of functions these nutrients perform in order to help control energy production in your body. In essence, however, the nutrients perform three basic functions relative to energy processes: (a) Some nutrients serve as an energy source, (b) some nutrients are needed to regulate the processes whereby energy is produced in the body, and (c) some nutrients are used to form the structure of and provide the growth and development for the various body tissues that produce energy (see Figure 3.1).

As the nutrients in food serve a wide variety of functions relative to energy production during exercise, it is no wonder that athletes throughout history have utilized a variety of foods in attempts to improve performance. In early Olympian times athletes devoured the meat from powerful animals, like lions. Thirty years ago they turned to honey and wheat-germ oil. Today the food technology industry has created for the athlete an array of such nutritional products as special amino acid mixtures recommended to increase muscle mass.

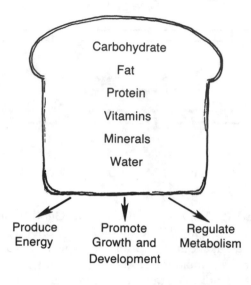

Carbohydrate

Fat

Protein

Vitamins

Minerals

Water

Produce
Energy

Promote
Growth and
Development

Regulate
Metabolism

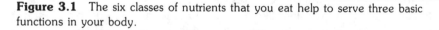

Figure 3.1 The six classes of nutrients that you eat help to serve three basic functions in your body.

Proper nutrition is essential for optimal sports performance. To be sure, if you are deficient in a nutrient that is important to energy production during exercise, your performance will suffer. A number of excellent experimental and clinical research studies have shown that such deficiencies will impair physiological functioning and physical performance. For example, one recent experimental study revealed a decrease in maximal oxygen uptake and aerobic endurance in athletes within a month after they were placed on a diet that induced a deficiency of several B vitamins. Recent clinical studies with female distance runners have also noted impaired endurance due to iron-deficiency anemia. In such cases, removing the deficiency by proper nutrition resulted in improved performance.

Generally speaking, if you are eating a varied diet containing wholesome foods you will not likely suffer from a nutrient deficiency that will impair athletic performance. Nevertheless, there is probably no sphere of nutrition where there are more myths and misconceptions than in athletic nutrition. As a consequence of these myths and misconceptions, many athletes, in an attempt to improve performance, are consuming substantial amounts of vitamins, minerals, amino acids, special forms of carbohydrates, and other nutritional products specifically marketed for athletes.

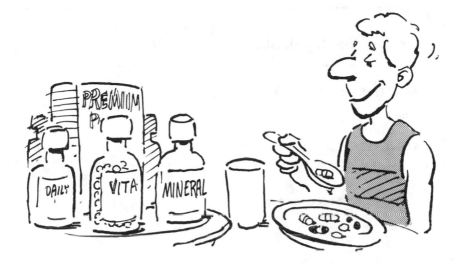

Six Classes of Nutrients

All the nutrients you need for optimal sports performance may be obtained from a well-balanced diet—this point will be stressed throughout this chapter. The nutrients you eat can be grouped into six different classes: *carbohydrates, fats, proteins, vitamins, minerals,* and *water.* In general, carbohydrates serve as a source of energy. Fats provide energy too, but are also part of the structure of most cells. Protein has a variety of roles: It is necessary for tissue formation, growth, and development; it is necessary for the formation of enzymes to regulate energy production; and, under certain conditions, it may be used as an energy source. Vitamins serve primarily to regulate a variety of metabolic processes by working with enzymes. Many minerals also are involved in the regulation of metabolism, but some contribute to the structure of your body as well. Finally, water comprises most of your body weight and helps to regulate a variety of body processes. Table 3.1 presents the nutrients currently believed to be essential for life.

Although all nutrients serve one or more of the three basic functions relative to energy production, a number of specific nutrients are especially important to these energy functions during exercise, when the rate of energy production is increased. For example, carbohydrates are a prime energy source in the muscle, iron is essential to transport adequate oxygen to the muscle cell, and protein serves as the foundation for the formation of muscle tissue.

TABLE 3.1
ESSENTIAL NUTRIENTS FOR HUMANS

CARBOHYDRATES
Fiber

FATS (ESSENTIAL FATTY ACIDS)
Linoleic fatty acid

PROTEINS (ESSENTIAL AMINO ACIDS)
Isoleucine

Leucine

Lysine

Methionine

Phenylalanine

Threonine

Tryptophan

Valine

Histidine (for children, but not adults)

VITAMINS

Water-Soluble	**Fat-Soluble**
Thiamine (B_1)	A (retinol)
Riboflavin (B_2)	D (calciferol)
Niacin	E (tocopherol)
Pyridoxine (B_6)	K
Pantothenic acid	
Folacin	
B_{12}	
Biotin	
Ascorbic acid (C)	

TABLE 3.1 (Cont.)

MINERALS

Major	Trace	
Calcium	Chromium	Molybdenum
Chloride	Cobalt	Nickel
Magnesium	Copper	Selenium
Phosphorus	Fluorine	Silicon
Potassium	Iodine	Tin
Sodium	Iron	Vanadium
Sulfur	Manganese	Zinc

WATER

In this chapter we will look at many of the nutrients that play important roles in energy production during exercise. The theoretical basis for the nutrient as an ergogenic aid will be presented first, followed by a synthesis of the available research relative to its effectiveness, and, finally, a general recommendation to the athlete.

Carbohydrates

Theoretical Basis

The major function of carbohydrates in the human body is to serve as a source of energy. In order to understand their role in the development of fatigue during exercise, let us look first at what happens in the body to the carbohydrates that you eat.

Dietary Carbohydrates, Glucose, and Glycogen.   Dietary carbohydrates come in a variety of forms, often collectively known as *sugars* and *starches*. *Glucose* and *fructose* are two of the most basic simple sugars and are found naturally in many fruits. *Sucrose*, or common table sugar, is also classified as a simple sugar, but is actually a combination of glucose and fructose. Starches, such as grains and vegetables, are long chains of glucose molecules. *Glucose polymers* are special forms of starch we shall discuss later. In the digestive process and through liver metabolism, the vast majority of the carbohydrates you consume are converted into glucose. Thus, after you have consumed a meal rich in carbohydrates the level of glucose in your blood will increase. Blood glucose is commonly known as blood sugar. An increased blood glucose level will stimulate the release of *insulin*, a hormone, from your pancreas. Insulin will then facilitate the transport of glucose from the blood into the various tissues in the body, most notably the liver and the muscles, where it will be converted to its storage form, glycogen. If carbohydrates are consumed in excess of your needs, they will be stored as fat. The processes just described are depicted in Figure 3.2.

The levels of blood glucose, liver glycogen, and muscle glycogen may have important roles in the development of fatigue. Blood glucose is the primary energy source for the central nervous system, including the brain. If your blood sugar drops to a very low level, a condition known as *hypoglycemia*, the brain may not function properly and you may experience symptoms of weakness and fatigue. Blood glucose may also be transported to the muscles, where it may be used for energy production during exercise.

Liver glycogen provides a reservoir of glucose that is released into the blood in time of need. Normally there is only a small amount of glucose in your blood, so it must be replaced as it is used. As your blood sugar level falls, the liver glycogen breaks down into glucose, which is released into the blood to help maintain normal levels.

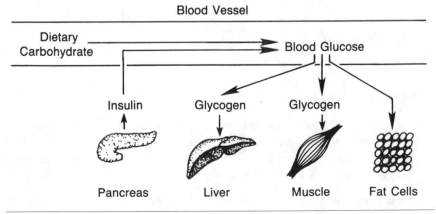

Figure 3.2   Dietary carbohydrate is converted into blood glucose. High blood glucose levels stimulate the pancreas to release insulin, which helps transport glucose into the muscles and other tissues. For athletes, adequate stores of muscle glycogen, liver glycogen, and blood glucose are important.

Carbohydrate Use During Exercise.   Muscle glycogen is utilized to regenerate ATP in order for muscle contraction to continue. As noted in the previous chapter, the glycogen in the FT muscle fibers is the only fuel source for the lactic acid energy system used in intense anaerobic-type exercise. Furthermore, the glycogen in the ST muscle fiber is the preferred fuel for the oxygen energy system during high-level aerobic exercise.

The rate at which you use your muscle glycogen stores depends primarily upon how intensely you exercise. If you perform high-speed anaerobic exercise, you will use the glycogen in your FT fibers at a fast rate. As mentioned in the last chapter, this type of exercise may result in the rapid production of lactic acid that may lead to the early development of fatigue.

During aerobic exercise you will use a combination of muscle glycogen and fats as the energy sources in your ST muscle fibers. However, as you increase the intensity of your aerobic exercise you will begin to use proportionally more glycogen than fats because glycogen is a more efficient fuel. In essence, you obtain about 7 percent more energy when you use glycogen instead of fats. Depending on how well trained you are, you may be able to use the muscle glycogen in your ST muscle fibers and exercise at a high percentage of your maximal oxygen uptake without accumulating excess lactic acid, and thus may continue to exercise for a prolonged period of time.

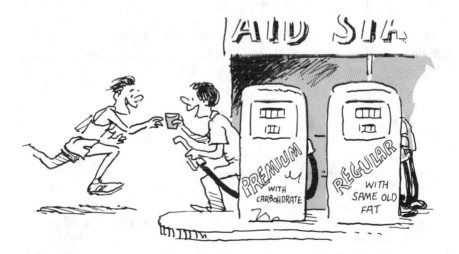

Carbohydrates and Fatigue.   Unfortunately, you cannot normally store large amounts of glycogen in your muscles, so glycogen may last for only an hour or so of high-level aerobic exercise. As your muscle glycogen stores deplete during prolonged exercise, your blood helps to deliver glucose from the liver to your muscles to allow you to maintain your energy production at a given level. However, as the liver glycogen stores are also limited, they will eventually be unable to provide adequate glucose to the blood.

Inadequate carbohydrate stores in the body may contribute to fatigue in several different ways. The athletic events most affected are those that depend on high levels of endurance—either intermittent bursts of speed over prolonged periods of time, as in games like soccer and basketball, or prolonged aerobic events such as the 26.2-mile (42.2-kilometer) marathon.

The soccer player is constantly on the run for 90 minutes or more, usually interspersing periods of high-speed, intense sprinting with recovery periods of less intense jogging. During the intense sprinting the FT muscle fibers are using glycogen rapidly; consequently, during the latter part of the second half of the match the glycogen content in these fibers might be too low to support sustained levels of high-speed running. This inability to maintain an optimal speed throughout the game is one example of fatigue.

In a marathon there are several possible causes of fatigue. First, the decrease in your blood glucose may deprive the brain of its primary energy source and result in sensations of weakness. Second, the depletion of glycogen in the ST muscle fibers toward the end of the race may have several effects. Your ST fibers will now need to use fat as an energy source, and because your oxygen energy system cannot produce ATP as rapidly from fat as it can from glycogen, your pace will slow down. If you want to maintain your pace you will need to recruit some FT muscle fibers to maintain an adequate rate of ATP production. As it appears to take mental energy to activate the FT fibers, maintaining your pace is psychologically stressful and fatiguing.

As is probably obvious, the basic theory underlying the use of carbohydrates as an ergogenic aid involves the maintenance of adequate blood glucose and muscle glycogen levels during prolonged bouts of exercise.

Research Findings

Literally thousands of studies have been conducted over the past century regarding the influence of the intake of carbohydrate on various aspects of athletic performance. German research in the year 1900 revealed that during exercise carbohydrate is a more efficient fuel than fat. Researchers in Scandinavia about 50 years ago discovered that diets high in carbohydrate would prolong exercise endurance capacity better than a normal balanced diet or a high-fat diet. Unfortunately, this knowledge was not usually applied to sports and the diet of the athlete for many years remained high in protein content.

However, in the 1960s and 1970s increasing research attention was devoted to the science of sport. The application of the electron microscope, the advent of the muscle-biopsy procedure, the ability to rapidly monitor oxygen consumption and blood composition changes, and other high-technology applications to sport, combined with an increasing number of scientists channeling their energies into sports science, led to a phenomenal increase in the number of research studies designed to improve athletic performance. Within these studies the area of nutrition was of prime interest, particularly the role of dietary carbohydrates.

In order to use carbohydrates as a means to improve athletic performance during competition, the major focus of the research was to develop feeding techniques to (a) help prevent the development of hypoglycemia, (b) help maintain an optimal supply of carbohydrate to the active muscles, and (c) maximize the storage of carbohydrate in the body prior to the event. Researchers have investigated a variety of issues, including the specific types of athletic events that would benefit from these feeding techniques, the most appropriate type and amount of carbohydrate to use, the most appropriate time to ingest the carbohydrate, and a special procedure known as *carbohydrate loading*.

Type of Athletic Event.   In general, research has shown that special carbohydrate-feeding techniques are not useful in athletic events of short duration (an hour or less). In such events the athlete, if rested for a day or two and on an average balanced diet, should have enough carbohydrate stored in the body to sustain energy production for this amount of time. Under such circumstances, adding extra carbohydrate to the body is analogous to putting an extra gallon of gas into a car to make it go faster on a short ride. On the other hand, carbohydrate feedings may be an effective ergogenic aid for those athletic activities characterized by prolonged endurance. Examples, as noted previously, include prolonged bouts of sustained aerobic exercise, such as marathon running, or prolonged exercise involving intermittent bursts of anaerobic energy production, such as soccer matches. Research has suggested that a selective depletion of glycogen from the ST muscle fibers may hamper performance in prolonged aerobic endurance exercise, whereas a depletion of glycogen from the FT muscle fibers may impair anaerobic energy production in the latter stages of a prolonged athletic contest.

Type and Amount of Carbohydrate.   Research has been conducted with a variety of types of carbohydrate, including glucose, fructose, sucrose, and glucose polymers, either alone or in combination, such as fructose and a glucose polymer together. These carbohydrates are usually administered in a liquid form, although solid carbohydrates have also been studied. As all carbohydrate forms must be converted into glucose in the body before they can enter the muscle cell, it appears logical that glucose would be the best form to consume.

However, there are several considerations that may dictate the choice of which type of carbohydrate to consume prior to competition. For example, of these carbohydrates, glucose will produce the greatest insulin response and fructose will produce the least. An exaggerated insulin response might lead to a reactive hypoglycemia and feelings of generalized weakness. Some early research has suggested that glucose consumption 30 to 45 minutes prior to exercise will lead to an increased utilization of muscle glycogen stores and possible impairment in endurance performance. However, several recent studies have failed to confirm this finding.

Another consideration may be the influence of the carbohydrate on the rate at which fluids leave the stomach. Research suggests that glucose polymers do not restrict gastric emptying of fluids as much as glucose does, although some recent research suggests that the difference may not be too important in endurance exercise. Another concern is the possible development of *gastrointestinal distress*, such as diarrhea, due to delayed absorption of some of the carbohydrate compounds from the intestine. Some studies have reported high incidence rates of gastrointestinal distress with fructose, possibly due to the fact that its rate of absorption from the intestines is slow.

However, it is important to note that most studies show there generally appears to be little difference between the various forms of carbohydrate (when consumed in the proper manner) in their ability to prevent hypoglycemia, to maintain optimal utilization of glucose by the muscle cells, and to improve performance in endurance events.

Timing of Intake.   The timing of the carbohydrate intake may be important for the athlete both in competition and in training. The following is a summary of the research concerning carbohydrate feedings prior to, during, and following exercise.

If carbohydrate is to be consumed 30 to 60 minutes prior to exercise, the best form to take is probably fructose, as its absorption is delayed somewhat and does not produce a large insulin response. As previously noted, some—but not all—research on glucose feedings taken 30 to 60 minutes before exercise revealed an exaggerated insulin response, a reactive hypoglycemia, an increased utilization of muscle glycogen, and a decrease in performance capacity in an endurance exercise task.

However, research suggests that it may be better to consume carbohydrates within 5 minutes or so of the start of competition. It takes time for the carbohydrate to be emptied from the stomach, absorbed through the intestines, and transported by the blood to the pancreas to stimulate insulin release. On the other hand, exercise may lead to the rapid release of certain hormones, particularly adrenalin, that help to suppress the release of insulin and actually contribute to a rise in the blood glucose level.

Research has also revealed that carbohydrate ingested prior to or during exercise may be used as a source of muscle energy within roughly 10 to 20 minutes. When you are performing an endurance event at about 60 to 70 percent of your maximal oxygen uptake, the rate at which the muscles are using glycogen is high. Unfortunately, your body cannot consume and absorb carbohydrate rapidly enough to replace your liver and muscle glycogen stores, so eventually these diminish and fatigue develops. However, the ingestion of carbohydrate sources will help to prevent the premature development of hypoglycemia and help to prolong the time that the muscles can use carbohydrate as an energy source, thus helping to improve performance. (You will not be able to run at a faster pace, but your ability to run at your optimal pace will be increased, leading to an overall faster time in endurance events.) Also, research with soccer players has suggested that the ingestion of carbohydrate sources might prevent the early development of fatigue in the later stages of a game, thus helping the players to maintain speed for a longer time.

Many laboratory studies have supported these results, but let's look at a recent field study with 12 world-class athletes. These bicyclists completed three 55-mile time trials about a week apart. The time trials consisted of six loops on a course slightly longer than 9 miles. The bicyclists were evenly paced for the first 5 loops, then went all-out for the last. In the first trial they consumed artificially sweetened water, in the second trial they consumed a 7 percent glucose-polymer solution, and in the third trial they had a 7 percent glucose-polymer-fructose solution. When they consumed water only, the athletes performed more than 2 minutes slower than they did when they took the carbohydrate solutions.

On a daily basis, carbohydrate intake following competition or hard training workouts may help to facilitate recovery. Some research has suggested that consuming carbohydrate immediately, or at least within 2 hours, after endurance competition or intense training will facilitate the storage of glycogen in the muscle. A diet high in carbohydrates is very important for the endurance athlete who trains intensely on a day-to-day basis.

Carbohydrate Loading.   Carbohydrate loading, also known as *glycogen loading* or *muscle glycogen supercompensation*, is a special technique developed over the years primarily for long-distance runners and cross-country skiers, but which may also be useful for such other endurance athletes as bicyclists and swimmers. Moreover, the basic theory and techniques underlying carbohydrate loading, or *carbo loading*, may also be appropriate for athletes in other sports, such as tennis, field hockey, and soccer, who may be competing in several games in a day or two, as might happen in tournament competition.

As you can infer from its name, the basic purpose of carbohydrate loading is to increase the stores of carbohydrate in the body, primarily the muscle and liver glycogen levels. Modification of exercise training and diet are both important. Although several techniques have been used over the years, the currently recommended procedure for trained endurance athletes is to taper the intensity of exercise training for a week or so prior to competition. Before this tapering phase, or about 7 to 10 days prior to competition, an endurance athlete might want to perform a moderately long exercise task, whereas a soccer player might play several consecutive practice games with frequent bursts of speed. However, recent research has noted that these exercise tasks should not be exhausting. During the tapering phase the athlete eats a limited amount of carbohydrate, then shifts to a high carbohydrate diet for several days prior to competition. Research has shown that such a technique will increase both the liver and muscle glycogen stores, with muscle biopsies showing more than twice the amount of glycogen present than during a noncarbohydrate-loaded condition. Research also supports the finding that carbohydrate loading will improve performance in prolonged endurance events. As with carbohydrate intake before or during performance, carbohydrate loading will not help you run faster during the early stages of an endurance event, but you will be able to maintain an optimal pace for a longer period of time.

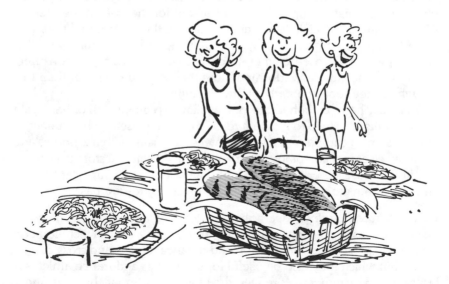

Recommendations

Most athletes do not consume enough carbohydrate on a day-to-day basis. Thus, a basic recommendation for all athletes, particularly endurance athletes, is a diet that stresses the complex carbohydrates. Approximately

60 to 70 percent of the daily dietary calories should be derived from carbohydrates within the basic four food groups. Good sources within the bread and cereal group include whole-grain breads and cereals, rice, and pasta such as macaroni and spaghetti. Beans are actually classified in the meat group due to their high protein content, but are also very high in carbohydrate. Under certain conditions they may also provide a beneficial jet-propulsion effect. In the milk group, skim milk is an excellent source of carbohydrate, as are most foods in the fruit and vegetable group. A balanced diet containing many of these high-carbohydrate foods will help to insure adequate body reserves of liver and muscle glycogen for sustained high-intensity training.

For most athletes, this basic diet coupled with a tapering period will provide adequate liver and muscle glycogen stores for competition in events of sustained or intermittent exercise for an hour or so. Athletes competing for longer periods of time, such as 2 hours or more, may want to consider both carbohydrate loading and carbohydrate intake just prior to and during performance.

Carbohydrate Loading.   The full program of carbohydrate loading may be recommended for major competitions, such as a marathon or a 2- or 3-day soccer tournament at the end of a season. Table 3.2 presents a recommended format for a 1-week carbohydrate-loading regimen. The depletion phase, as noted before, is characterized by prolonged exercise to reduce

---

TABLE 3.2
A RECOMMENDED CARBOHYDRATE-LOADING REGIMEN

Day 1	Moderately long exercise bout (should not be exhaustive)
Day 2	Mixed diet; moderate carbohydrate intake; tapering exercise
Day 3	Mixed diet; moderate carbohydrate intake; tapering exercise
Day 4	Mixed diet; moderate carbohydrate intake; tapering exercise
Day 5	High-carbohydrate diet; tapering exercise
Day 6	High-carbohydrate diet; tapering exercise or rest
Day 7	High-carbohydrate diet; tapering exercise or rest
Day 8	Competition

Note. The moderate carbohydrate intake should approximate 200 to 300 grams of carbohydrate per day; the high carbohydrate intake should approximate 500 to 600 grams of carbohydrate per day.

the amount of glycogen in the muscles and liver. The exercise task should not be exhausting in nature. The exercise task is followed by 3 days of tapering exercise and moderate carbohydrate intake and then 3 days of tapering exercise or rest and high carbohydrate intake (approximately 500 to 600 grams of carbohydrates per day).

Table 3.3 presents some guidelines to the gram carbohydrate content of various high-carbohydrate foods. These foods should be stressed in the daily diet along with about 6 to 8 ounces of lean meat, poultry, or fish to guarantee adequate high-quality protein intake. Skim milk is also a good source of high-quality protein. The following foods consumed in the main meals and snacks throughout the day will provide over 500 grams of carbohydrate:

6 slices of bread	2 bagels
2 cups cooked pasta	1 cup dry cereal
2 glasses skim milk	1/2 cup baked beans
2 bananas	1 cup orange juice
1 baked potato	1 cup pineapple juice
1 apple	1/4 cup dried peaches
6 gingersnaps	1 ounce pretzels

A good way to tell if you have increased your body carbohydrate stores is to weigh yourself daily during the week. When the carbohydrate is stored in your muscles as glycogen it binds excess water with it. Thus, depending on your present level of muscle glycogen, your body weight will *probably* increase several pounds during the 3 days of carbohydrate loading. Your active muscles may also feel somewhat tight due to the increased amount of glycogen and water in the muscles.

Carbohydrate Intake Before or During Exercise.   If you plan to consume carbohydrates immediately before and during prolonged endurance exercise, one recommended procedure is to consume a rather highly concentrated solution (about 35 to 40 percent) approximately 5 minutes prior to the event and less-concentrated solutions (about 5 to 10 percent) at regular intervals during the event. You should have about 40 to 50 grams prior to the event and about 15 to 20 grams *every* 20 minutes or so during the event. The dry polymer mixed in water is an easy method to use. Ultradistance athletes may wish to consume higher concentrations during the event.

The amount of carbohydrate in commercial sport drinks varies. The most popular brand, Gatorade, is a 5 to 6 percent solution of glucose. Others may be as low as 1 percent or as high as 10 percent. If you want to try

TABLE 3.3
GRAMS OF CARBOHYDRATE
IN THE BASIC FOOD EXCHANGES

STARCHY VEGETABLES, BREADS, AND CEREALS— 15 GRAMS CARBOHYDRATE PER SERVING

One Serving:

1/2 cup dry breakfast cereals	1 small baked potato
1/2 cup cooked breakfast cereals	1/2 bagel
1/2 cup cooked grits	1/2 English muffin
1/3 cup cooked rice	1 slice bread
1/2 cup cooked pasta	3/4 ounce pretzels
1/4 cup baked beans	6 saltine crackers
1/2 cup corn	2 four-inch-diameter pancakes
1/2 cup beans	2 taco shells

VEGETABLES—5 GRAMS CARBOHYDRATE PER SERVING

One Serving:

1/2 cup cooked vegetables

1 cup raw vegetables

1/2 cup vegetable juice

Examples: carrots, green beans, broccoli, cauliflower, onions, spinach, tomatoes, vegetable juice

FRUITS—15 GRAMS CARBOHYDRATE PER SERVING

One Serving:

1/2 cup fresh fruit	12 cherries
1/2 cup fruit juice	1/2 grapefruit
1/4 cup dried fruit	1 nectarine
1 small apple	1 orange
4 apricots	1 peach
1/2 banana	1-1/4 cup watermelon

TABLE 3.3 (Cont.)

MILK – 12 GRAMS CARBOHYDRATE PER SERVING

One Serving:

1 cup skim milk

8 ounces plain low-fat yogurt

SWEETS – 15 GRAMS CARBOHYDRATE PER SERVING

One Serving:

1/2 slice cake	1/2 cup ice cream
2 small cookies	1/4 cup sherbet
3 gingersnaps	

Note. Adapted from *Exchange Lists for Meal Planning* by the American Diabetes Association and American Dietetic Association, 1986, Chicago: American Dietetic Association.

preparing your own sport drink, dry glucose polymers are available in many sporting goods stores. Two popular brands are Gatorlode (not Gatorade) and Exceed. To make a solution of a given percentage you need to put a certain amount (dry ounces) of the polymer powder into a certain amount (fluid ounces) of water. A measuring cup may be used to measure ounces. Two ounces of dry powder in a quart of water (32 ounces) will produce a solution of about 6 percent (2/32 = 0.0625). If you put one level tablespoon (0.5 ounce) of the polymer in a glass of water (8 ounces), you will have about a 6 to 7 percent solution (0.5/8 = 0.0625). Figure 3.3 illustrates how to make a 6 percent, a 20 percent, and a 35 percent solution using a quart of water for each. You may also follow the directions usually found on the commercial products.

Carbohydrate and Water Intake.   As noted later in this chapter, water intake is important for maintaining proper body temperature for athletes who compete and train in warm environmental temperatures. Findings from early research suggest that the carbohydrate content in fluids should be less than 2.5 percent in order to not impair water absorption into the body. However, the focus of this research was on how carbohydrate concentration affects the rate at which fluids empty from the stomach, not on the rate at which they are absorbed into the body from the intestines. More

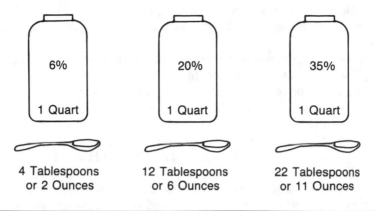

Figure 3.3 How to make a 6, 20, or 35 percent glucose-polymer solution.

recent research suggests that carbohydrate concentrations of 5 to 10 percent do not appear to impair water absorption or temperature regulation during prolonged exercise in the heat. Thus, the endurance athlete may use the recommended procedures even when exercising in warm temperatures.

Legal, Ethical, and Medical Considerations. The use of carbohydrate supplementation as an ergogenic aid does not appear to pose any legal, ethical, or medical problems, although diabetic athletes should consult their physicians regarding any possible complications.

   As with most legal and safe ergogenic aids discussed in this book, the athlete should experiment with the aid in training and practice before trying it in competition. For example, high concentrations of fructose and the glucose polymers may lead to diarrhea in some individuals, which could be a debilitating experience during a competitive athletic event.

Fats

Theoretical Basis

Dietary fats play a number of different physiological roles in the body, but one of the most significant is to serve as a fuel for the oxygen energy system. As noted in the previous section, fat is a less efficient fuel than carbohydrate; fat produces less ATP per liter of oxygen consumed and produces it at a slower rate. During rest and low-intensity exercise the energy demand is not that great, so fat may provide 50 to 60 percent of the energy needs. However, as the exercise intensity increases, the muscles begin to use increasing amounts of carbohydrate and proportionately lesser amounts of fat.

As you become better trained your muscles make several adaptations to help improve your performance. In essence, they develop a greater ability to use both carbohydrates and fats as sources of energy during exercise. The ability to oxidize carbohydrates at a faster rate allows you to produce ATP more rapidly and thus helps improve your overall speed. For example, in running you may maintain a mile pace of 6 minutes, 30 seconds instead of 7 minutes. The ability to oxidize fats at a faster rate allows you to substitute fat for carbohydrate as an energy source at a given speed. For example, the energy needed to run a 7-minute mile before training may necessitate 80 percent from carbohydrate and 20 percent from fat; however, after training it may be reduced to 65 percent from carbohydrate and 35 percent from fat. Some highly trained athletes may derive over 50 percent of their energy needs from fat even when performing fairly-high-intensity exercise. Thus, by using proportionately more fat, training helps you to spare some of your carbohydrate stores.

Figure 3.4 presents a schematic of fat as an energy source during exercise. Fat is stored as *triglycerides* (compounds containing fatty acids and glycerol, a type of alcohol) in both the muscle and the adipose tissue. During exercise the muscle triglycerides break down into free fatty acids (FFA) and glycerol, the FFA eventually being processed into the *mitochondria* (energy-producing factories in the cells) to provide ATP via the oxygen energy system. The glycerol is released into the blood for transport to the liver for further metabolism. The adipose tissue throughout the body, under the influence of hormones such as *epinephrine* (adrenalin), also breaks down its triglycerides, with the FFA traveling via the blood to the muscles and the glycerol going to the liver.

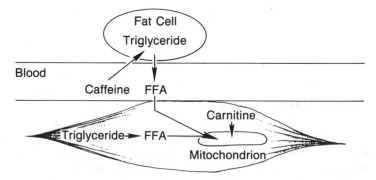

Figure 3.4   Fat can be used as an energy source during exercise. Triglycerides in fat cells may release free fatty acids (FFA) into the blood for transport to the muscle. Supplies in the muscle may also be used. Caffeine and carnitine are two ergogenic aids used in attempts to improve the use of fats during exercise. Their roles are discussed in later chapters.

The preferred fuel for high-intensity exercise is carbohydrate, but the liver and muscles have a limited capacity to store carbohydrate in the form of glycogen and may become depleted in very prolonged athletic events— for example, in running events over 20 miles. On the other hand, the body stores fat in a very compact form, and these fat stores would provide the average individual with enough energy to run over 800 miles. Consequently, it may be advantageous for some endurance athletes to optimize the utilization of fat as an energy source in order to spare enough liver and muscle glycogen for the later stages of a contest.

Research Findings

The effect of high-fat diets on athletic performance has been studied in a variety of ways; the results almost universally support the conclusion that such diets are actually detrimental to performance in endurance exercise. For example, many of the studies that investigated the relationship between high-carbohydrate diets and physical performance compared the effect to performance when the subjects were on a high-fat diet. Invariably, physical performance was worse on the high-fat diets.

In one study, five well-trained bicyclists subsisted for nearly a month on a high-fat diet, with over 80 percent of their calories coming from fat. Although the cyclists were able to adapt to the diet and to perform effectively at about 60 to 65 percent of their maximal oxygen uptake, the principal investigators in this study did not recommend this type of diet for endurance athletes. Moreover, other research has shown that such diets lead to decreases in power.

Recommendations

Diets high in fat are not recommended for athletes for several reasons. First, they will not improve but may actually impair athletic performance. Furthermore, such diets may pose significant health risks to some individuals by increasing the possibility of developing several chronic diseases, such as cancer and coronary heart disease.

On the other hand, various agents have been used in attempts to mobilize FFA during exercise so that they might be used preferentially as a fuel and therefore help spare the utilization of muscle glycogen. As noted in Figure 3.4, caffeine may be utilized to facilitate the breakdown of triglycerides and the release of FFA from the adipose tissue or from within the muscle cell, whereas carnitine is needed to transport FFA from the cytoplasm into the mitochondria. Caffeine will be discussed in the chapter on pharmacological aids; carnitine will be covered in the physiological aids chapter.

Protein and Amino Acid Supplements

Theoretical Basis

Protein is one of your most essential nutrients. The protein in your diet is broken down by the digestive process into 20 different amino acids. These amino acids are absorbed into your bloodstream, transported to the liver for further metabolism, and then distributed by the blood to all cells of the body for the formation of proteins specific to the functions of the different cells.

Protein Functions and RDA.
Protein serves all three functions of nutrients. First, protein is the primary nutrient involved in growth, development, and repair of all body tissues. For example, although your muscle tissues consist of approximately 72 percent water, 22 of the remaining 28 percent is protein. Protein is the structural basis for all body tissues. Second, protein is essential for the regulation of metabolism. All metabolic reactions in your body are controlled by *enzymes*, and all enzymes are formed from protein. And third, although protein is not a primary source of energy, it may be used for such purposes under certain conditions. As a matter of fact, the use of body-protein stores, such as muscle, as a source of energy takes precedence over the other two functions when caloric intake is inadequate, as in starvation. In such cases, as known to many young men in the sport of wrestling, performance may deteriorate due to loss of muscle mass.

Your body is continually synthesizing new protein and excreting the waste products of protein metabolism. One element found in protein that is not contained in carbohydrate and fat is nitrogen, but in order for nitrogen to be stored in the body, it must be part of protein. Nitrogen itself is not stored in the body, so the residue left from protein breakdown is excreted in the urine. In order for your body to function at an optimal level, the nitrogen you excrete needs to be replaced. If you replace what you excrete, you are said to be in *nitrogen balance*, or *protein balance*. If you gain weight through weight training, you are usually in a state of *positive protein balance*. Weight loss through such techniques as starvation-type diets results in a *negative protein balance*.

In the United States, the *recommended dietary allowance* (RDA) for each nutrient has been developed by a group of nutrition scientists; the allowance is designed to meet the nutritional needs of all healthy individuals. The protein RDA is different for young children, adolescents, and adults.

Because children and adolescents are in a stage of growth and development they need a positive protein balance, whereas the normal adult needs only to maintain normal protein balance. The sedentary adolescent requires about 0.45 grams of protein per pound of body weight on a daily basis, whereas the sedentary adult needs only about 0.36 grams per pound. Thus, the RDA for a 154-pound adolescent is about 70 grams per day, but an adult with the same body weight needs only about 56 grams.

Protein and Exercise.   Exercise training exerts a significant effect upon protein metabolism in the body. As mentioned earlier, exercise training produces a variety of changes in the body that help to facilitate the production and utilization of energy. In some way, exercise training stimulates the nucleus of the cell to increase the production of proteins important for energy utilization. The type of protein that is produced is specific to the exercise stimulus. For example, weight training will stimulate an increase in the amount of *contractile muscle protein*, so the muscle may experience a significant increase in size and strength. On the other hand, aerobic endurance exercise will stimulate the formation of *mitochondrial protein* (the mitochondria are the energy powerhouses of the cell) and *oxidative enzyme proteins*, which will improve the ability of the muscle to produce ATP via the oxygen energy system, but the size of the muscle itself will not increase. Under conditions of low muscle glycogen stores, prolonged aerobic endurance exercise may also use protein sources in the body for energy; however, these protein sources are not as efficient as muscle glycogen.

So, depending on the type of exercise training, dietary protein may be used to support muscle growth, to produce enzymes necessary for energy metabolism, or to serve as a source of energy. Manufacturers of nutrient supplements for athletes have capitalized on this situation. In particular, protein and amino acid supplements have been marketed for bodybuilders, weight lifters, and power athletes as a means of maximizing muscle growth and strength gains. One amino acid supplement is advertised to be more effective as a means of increasing muscle mass and body weight than the most powerful anabolic steroid. Protein supplements have also been marketed specifically for endurance athletes, with the suggestion that they improve endurance capacity.

There is some debate among investigators in sports nutrition whether or not athletes need additional protein in the diet. One point of view suggests that athletes need obtain only the RDA for protein of 0.36 to 0.45 grams per pound of body weight, as the RDA itself generally provides more protein than is necessary. On the other hand, other investigators recommend amounts ranging from 0.9 to 1.4 grams per pound.

Research Findings

You should be aware that the research studies reported in advertisements for protein and amino acid supplements, particularly in magazines for bodybuilders and strength athletes, are not reliable sources of information. In most cases these "research studies" are very poorly controlled and consist of personal testimonials. None of them have undergone the scientific scrutiny necessary to be published in reputable scientific journals, but are used to provide "scientific" support to enhance sales. On the other hand, some well-designed studies have been published in sports science journals and provide us with sound information about the protein needs of athletes in training.

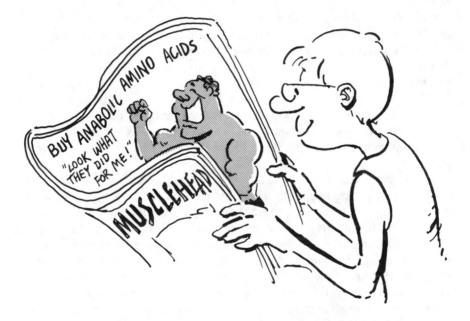

Protein and Endurance Athletes.   Research with endurance athletes has revealed that under some conditions, particularly when body stores of carbohydrate are low, protein may account for 5 to 10 percent of the energy needed during exercise. As mentioned previously, carbohydrate in the form of blood glucose is essential for optimal functioning of the brain, so the blood glucose level needs to be maintained at normal levels during exercise. One means to help maintain a normal blood glucose level is to convert protein into glucose. This is accomplished in the body when muscle protein breaks down to form *alanine*, an amino acid that is released into the blood and travels to the liver for conversion into glucose. The glucose is then released into the blood (see Figure 3.5). When carbohydrate levels in the body are low, as is the case in the later stages of prolonged exercise, this process appears to be accelerated. This again reinforces the importance of carbohydrate in the diet of the athlete, for carbohydrate helps to spare the utilization of muscle protein.

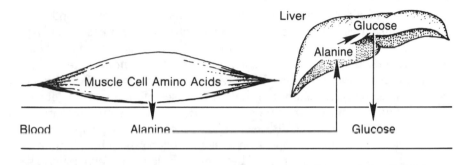

Figure 3.5   Muscle protein may be broken down and used for energy production under some conditions. One mechanism is the glucose-alanine cycle, explained in the text.

If we assume a high value (10 percent) of the energy cost during exercise is being contributed by protein, total protein spent would be approximately 25 grams for the endurance athlete who exercises strenuously for 60 to 90 minutes per day. This athlete may also lose some protein in sweat and urine, but this amount, about 5 to 7 grams per day on days with a strenuous workout, is relatively low. Thus, the estimation of the total daily protein cost of exercise for the endurance athlete is about 30 to 35 grams.

Virtually no research exists on the use of protein or amino acid supplements as a means of improving performance in endurance athletes who are in protein balance. Some early Japanese research found that athletes in training on low-protein diets, less than 0.23 grams of protein per pound of body weight, developed a condition known as *sports anemia* which could impair performance. However, athletes consuming about 0.45 grams per pound of body weight did not experience such problems.

Protein, Amino Acids, and Muscle Development.   Weight-training exercise in itself does not appear to use protein as a fuel for energy, but protein is necessary to synthesize new muscle tissue. Several research studies support the need for additional protein during weight-training programs to increase muscle mass. One well-designed study compared two groups of men involved in weight training; one group received 0.36 to 0.64 grams of protein per pound of body weight daily and a second group received 1.1 to 1.3 grams per pound. The second group did gain more weight than the first, and the gains were suggested to be in lean muscle mass, not body fat. However, there were no significant differences between the groups relative to strength gains or other physiological measures of performance. One recent study did show improvement in strength when elite weight lifters increased their daily protein intake from 1.1 to 1.6 grams per pound, but the study was poorly designed and the results could be attributed to increased intensity of weight training.

Amino acid supplements have recently been advertised for strength athletes because they are said to provide a safe *anabolic*, or muscle-building, effect. The two most commonly used amino acids are *arginine* and *ornithine*. They are theorized to increase the levels of *growth hormone* (often called human growth hormone, or hGH), which has a potent anabolic effect. Some earlier research has noted that large doses of arginine, if injected, could stimulate growth hormone release. However, no sound research is currently available on the anabolic effects of these amino acid supplements on athletes. Moreover, findings from well-controlled research with animals involved in exercise training reveal that these supplements neither increase levels of growth hormone nor provide an anabolic effect.

As we shall see in a later chapter, drugs known as *anabolic steroids* have been utilized by athletes to increase muscle mass and strength, but these drugs may have some serious medical side effects.

Recommendations

It should be emphasized that athletes who consume a typical American diet and enough calories to maintain their body weight will obtain sufficient protein to maintain protein balance. But, in general, athletes involved in either strenuous weight training or strenuous aerobic endurance training may need slightly additional amounts of protein in their diet. Some investigators in the area of sports nutrition recommend a daily protein intake ranging from about 0.7 to 1.4 grams per pound of body weight. The lower levels have usually been applied to endurance athletes; the higher values have been suggested for strength athletes in weight training.

Let us look at some mathematics relative to protein intake. Table 3.4 presents some data relative to the daily protein requirements according to the recommendations just noted. At 0.7 grams of protein per pound of body weight, a 140-pound cross-country runner would need about 98 grams of protein per day and a 180-pound strength athlete at 1.4 grams of protein per pound of body weight would need a whopping 252 grams. Obtaining 98 grams should be no problem for the runner. If we assume he needs 20 calories per pound of body weight to meet his daily energy needs—as he expends many calories in training—then he should eat about 2800 calories per day. If 15 percent of these calories are derived from protein, a reasonable percentage, then 420 calories will come from protein

(2800 × .15). Because each gram of protein equals 4 calories, the runner will get about 105 grams of protein (420/4), which is more than enough to meet his recommended needs. However, the recommended amount for the strength athlete would necessitate a protein intake equivalent to approximately 30 percent of the daily calories. The number of calories per pound of body weight is only 18 because the strength athlete does not expend as many calories through exercise as the runner.

The point should be reemphasized here that most of the available evidence indicates that 0.7 grams per pound of body weight will satisfy the protein need of all athletes. The recommendations of investigators who have spent a lifetime working with protein nutrition support this evidence.

TABLE 3.4
DAILY PROTEIN CONTENT
TO MEET MINIMUM AND MAXIMUM SUGGESTIONS

	ENDURANCE ATHLETE	STRENGTH ATHLETE
Body weight in pounds	140	180
Recommended grams of protein/ pound	0.7	1.4
Recommended total grams protein/ day	98	252
Calories/pound of body weight/day	20	18
Total calories/day	2800	3240
Percent calories from protein	15	31
Calories derived from protein	420	1004
Calories/gram of protein	4	4
Grams of protein consumed daily	105	251

High-Protein Foods.   The general recommendation for athletes is to obtain the protein they need through nutritious foods. Although protein supplements marketed for athletes often contain high-quality protein, such as milk solids and soybean protein, they are usually very expensive. Consumption of high-quality protein foods that are low in fat will help guarantee proper protein nutrition. Table 3.5 presents the protein content per serving of the basic food exchanges, along with the number of calories per serving; the additional calories are derived from the carbohydrate and/or fat content in the food.

High-quality protein foods are found in the milk and meat exchanges. Unfortunately, milk and meat foods often contain substantial amounts of fat, so you must be careful to select those that contain as little fat as possible in order to restrict caloric intake. Fish, white meat of chicken and turkey, lowfat meats, and skim milk are excellent selections. Egg whites are pure protein with no fat. Lean meats contain about 50 percent of the calories as protein, skim milk is about 40 percent protein, vegetables contain about 30 percent, and starchy foods are about 15 percent. The average American diet consists of about 15 percent protein.

Medical Considerations. Although protein content in the diet of 15 to 20 percent or so of the daily calories does not pose any serious medical risks to most individuals, higher amounts may. Since excess protein cannot be stored in the body, the excess nitrogen must be excreted by the kidneys. There is some concern that high protein intakes may overstress the kidney, which is one reason why adequate fluid intake is important for individuals on high-protein diets. Also, substances known as *purines* are often found in protein foods, and when purines are metabolized in the body some of the waste products may collect in the joints, leading to *gout*, an arthritic condition.

Consuming large amounts of individual amino acids may cause interference with the absorption and metabolism of other amino acids in the body, thus interfering with normal physiological functions.

From a performance standpoint, excess protein intake may predispose the athlete to dehydration because body fluids may be used to help excrete the excess nitrogen. High-protein diets have also been shown to increase metabolic heat production. Thus, athletes on high-protein diets who compete in warm environments may be at a disadvantage relative to temperature regulation.

Vitamins

Theoretical Basis

Vitamins function in your body to regulate a wide variety of metabolic processes, and they work in different ways. Most vitamins, particularly those in the vitamin B complex, are needed to activate enzymes necessary for energy production and a host of other physiological functions (see Figure 3.6). Some vitamins, such as A, C, and E, serve as powerful *antioxidants*, helping to prevent undesired oxidation of cell membranes, such as the red blood cell. One vitamin, D, actually functions as a hormone

TABLE 3.5
**GRAMS OF PROTEIN
PER SERVING FOR BASIC FOOD EXCHANGES**

MILK – 8 GRAMS PER SERVING

One Serving:	Calories:
1 cup skim milk	90
1 cup plain low-fat yogurt	90

LEAN MEAT – 7 GRAMS PER SERVING

One Serving:	Calories:
1 ounce lean beef or pork	55
1 ounce chicken or turkey (no skin)	45
1 ounce fish, shrimp, lobster, tuna	40
1 ounce wild game	55
1 ounce diet cheese	55
2 large egg whites	35

**STARCHY VEGETABLES, BREADS, AND CEREALS – 3 GRAMS
PER SERVING**

One Serving:	Calories:
1/2 cup cooked or dry cereal	80
1/2 cup cooked pasta	80
1/3 cup cooked rice	80
1/2 bagel	80
1 slice bread	80
1 small baked potato	80
1/4 cup baked beans	80

VEGETABLES – 2 GRAMS PER SERVING

One Serving:	Calories:
1/2 cup cooked vegetables	25
1 cup raw vegetables	25

FRUITS – ABOUT 1 GRAM OR LESS PER SERVING

One Serving:	Calories:
1 small apple	60

Note. Adapted from *Exchange Lists for Meal Planning* by the American
Diabetes Association and American Dietetic Association, 1986, Chicago:
American Dietetic Association.

to regulate calcium metabolism. In relation to exercise, vitamins cannot be used as actual sources of energy, but they are essential to help release the energy from carbohydrate and fat, to help regulate proper functioning of the nervous system, and to guarantee optimal operation of the energy support systems.

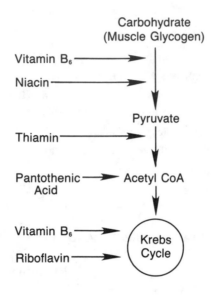

Figure 3.6 The B vitamins are important for the release of energy from carbohydrate in the muscle cell.

Each of the 13 vitamins has a number of specific functions in the body. Table 3.6 provides an overview of the major roles of each that may theoretically be important in exercise. The U.S. RDA or *estimated safe and adequate daily dietary intake (ESADDI)* is also presented for each vitamin; strictly speaking, the ESADDI is not the same as the RDA, but simply represents the amount of a nutrient believed by nutrition scientists to be safe and adequate in the diets of healthy Americans.

Although most nutritionists contend that a well-balanced diet will provide sufficient amounts of all vitamins, more than 40 percent of Americans above the age of 16 consume vitamin supplements, many believing that the typical American diet today is low in vitamin content. It is also a well-known fact that many athletes take vitamin supplements, possibly for the same reason, but also in the belief that athletes need more vitamins than sedentary individuals as a means of achieving optimal physical performance.

TABLE 3.6
**POSSIBLE ROLES OF VITAMINS
IMPORTANT DURING EXERCISE**

VITAMIN	U.S. RDA OR ESSADI	POSSIBLE ROLE
A (retinol)	5000 IU	Antioxidant; prevention of RBC damage
D (calciferol)	400 IU	Calcium transport in muscle
E (tocopherol)	15 IU	Antioxidant; prevention of RBC damage; promotion of aerobic energy production
K	.07 to .14 mg	None determined
B_1 (thiamine)	1.5 mg	Energy release from carbohydrate; formation of hemoglobin; proper nervous system functioning
B_2 (riboflavin)	1.7 mg	Energy release from carbohydrate and fat
Niacin	20 mg	Energy release from carbohydrate, both aerobic and anaerobic; blockage of release of FFA from adipose tissue
B_6 (pyridoxine)	2.2 mg	Energy release from carbohydrate; formation of hemoglobin and oxidative enzymes; proper nervous system functioning
B_{12}	.003 mg	RBC production
Folic acid	.4 mg	RBC production
Pantothenic acid	10 mg	Energy production from carbohydrate and fat
Biotin	.2 mg	Carbohydrate and fat synthesis
C (ascorbic acid)	60 mg	Antioxidant; increased absorption of iron; formation of epinephrine; promotion of aerobic energy production; formation of connective tissues

Note. IU = International Units; mg = milligrams.

Research Findings

The effect of vitamin nutrition on physical performance has been studied in a variety of ways. In some studies, subjects were placed on low-vitamin diets to create a vitamin deficiency. Other studies provided vitamin supplements to individuals with known deficiencies. Still others provided supplements to individuals who were on well-balanced diets and already obtaining the RDA for each vitamin.

Vitamin Deficiency and Sports Performance.   Although almost all vitamins have been studied in relation to physical performance, most of the research has focused on the B-complex vitamins and vitamins C and E. Vitamin C and especially the B-complex vitamins are water soluble, and thus are more readily excreted from the body. The body contains appreciable stores of the fat-soluble vitamins (A, D, E, K), so they are less likely to be depleted.

The results of the deficiency studies have shown that physical performance may decrease markedly, even within as short a period of time as 2 to 4 weeks, when the diet is low in the B vitamins. Both aerobic and anaerobic endurance capacity deteriorate, due presumably to either the body's inability to metabolize carbohydrate effectively or to the disruption of central nervous system functioning.

Research has also revealed that correcting a vitamin deficiency will improve physical performance. Many of these studies were conducted with children who had a poor diet due to environmental conditions in some countries. Several of the studies that actually created a vitamin deficiency in adults later gave supplements to the subjects to restore them to normal vitamin status. In such cases, physical performance did improve, but did not improve above the level of performance obtained prior to the deficiency state. In other words, vitamin supplementation simply restored physical performance back to normal levels, but contributed no additional benefits.

Vitamin Supplements and Sports Performance.   In general, research conducted over the past 50 years with well-nourished individuals has not revealed any beneficial effects of vitamin supplementation on physical performance. Early research did show some benefits, but the studies were poorly designed. In some studies from Poland, Russia, and other eastern European countries, the benefits may have been due to correction of a vitamin deficiency. The vast majority of contemporary research with well-designed studies reveals that vitamin supplementation—either single vitamins or multivitamin compounds—will not improve physical performance in well-nourished individuals.

A possible exception is the use of vitamin E at high altitudes. One well-designed study found that vitamin E may help to increase maximal oxygen uptake and reduce lactic acid production at a set exercise task (which suggests improved oxygen use in the muscle cells) at altitudes of 5,000 to 15,000 feet. Theoretically, the antioxidant effect of vitamin E could help prevent the oxidation of red-blood cell membranes caused by ozone at altitude. Also, some recent research has suggested that supplementation with several of the B vitamins (B_1, B_6, and B_{12}) may benefit fine motor control in pistol shooters. These findings are in contrast to the majority of the available research; thus, additional research is needed for verification.

Unfortunately, space does not permit a detailed presentation of all the research studies that have been conducted, but individual studies involving such endurance athletes as swimmers and cross-country runners have not revealed any improvement in laboratory measures of physical performance, such as maximal oxygen uptake, or field performances, such as distance runs, even after prolonged supplementation with large doses of several vitamins, particularly C, E, and several in the B complex. A very recent study with physically trained subjects revealed no improvement in maximal oxygen uptake, the anaerobic threshold, or endurance run performance after 4 months of supplementation with all vitamins (except K) and iron in amounts 10 times the RDA.

As a matter of fact, supplementation with niacin may impair performance in prolonged endurance events because niacin may block the release of FFA, which are important fuels as muscle glycogen levels become depleted.

Recommendations

Vitamins in Food.   The basic nutritional recommendation for all athletes is to consume a well-balanced diet including a wide variety of lean meats, low-fat milk products, whole-grain foods, and fresh fruits and vegetables. Such a diet will provide all of the essential vitamins for the athlete. For example, the following list of foods, although containing only about 1200 calories, meets the RDA for all vitamins.

2 cups fortified skim milk	1 medium carrot
4 slices whole-wheat bread	1 medium orange
3 ounces roasted chicken breast	1 stalk broccoli
2 ounces Grape Nuts cereal	1 tablespoon margarine
3 ounces tuna fish, in water	1/2 cup cauliflower

Some athletes, like wrestlers, distance runners, gymnasts, and ballet dancers, who are restricting food intake to lose weight for competition may not be getting an adequate dietary intake of vitamins (although, as just noted, careful food selection may provide adequate vitamin nutrition with only 1200 calories). Any athletes concerned that their diets are not providing an adequate amount of vitamins can ensure adequate vitamin nutrition simply by taking a daily vitamin tablet that contains the RDA. Avoid the expensive vitamin supplements marketed specifically for athletes and simply purchase the least expensive generic brand. There is essentially no difference between the two, except the cost.

Legal, Ethical, and Medical Considerations.   Unfortunately, some athletes may believe that because a vitamin deficiency might impair performance, extra vitamins may help to improve performance. Thus they consume prodigious amounts, or *megadoses*, sometimes over 1000 times the RDA. At present such intake is not considered illegal by sport-governing bodies, but it may pose some serious health risks.

A *vitamin megadose* is defined as a value 10 times the RDA, although it may be lower with vitamins A and D. This amount of most of the water-soluble vitamins does not usually pose any significant health risk because they are simply excreted in the urine. However, larger amounts of several may pose problems to susceptible individuals. For example, excess vitamin B_6 may cause neurological damage. Excessive amounts of vitamin C can lead to kidney stones.

Regarding the fat-soluble vitamins, vitamin E in amounts 10 times the RDA appears to be safe. Major health problems may be associated with megadoses of vitamins A and D. Prolonged intake of doses only 5 times the RDA for vitamin A may lead to weakness, headache, nausea, pain in the joints, and liver damage. Similar doses of vitamin D may cause nausea, vomiting, diarrhea, and damage to such soft tissues as the kidney, heart, and blood vessels, due to excess calcium deposits.

In short, megadose vitamins have no beneficial application to the average athlete and are potentially harmful.

Minerals

Theoretical Basis

Your body needs over 25 different minerals in order to support proper growth, development, and function. Minerals, like vitamins, may not be used by the body as a direct source of energy. A few minerals are used primarily for structural purposes. For example, about 98 percent of the calcium and 90 percent of the phosphorus stored in your body is used to form your bones and teeth. Of importance to you as an athlete is that all minerals are involved in the regulation of a variety of physiological processes.

Many of the minerals in your body function in a manner similar to vitamins, for they help to activate enzymes that control metabolic processes. These enzymes are often known as *metalloenzymes*. For example, zinc

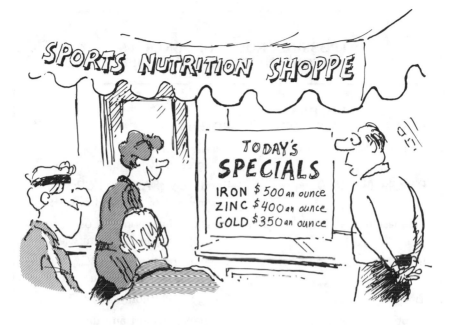

is a component of 60 or more enzymes, some of them involved in energy production within the muscle cell. Some minerals act as carrier systems, such as iron facilitating the transport of oxygen to the muscle cell. Others form *electrolytes*, or electrically charged particles called *ions*, in the body fluids. These electrolytes are used to create electrical energy necessary for the transmission of nerve impulses throughout the body, the initiation of muscle contraction, and a variety of other physiological functions.

Table 3.7 presents several of the key minerals in the body that have important roles relative to physical performance. The United States Recommended Daily Allowance (U.S. RDA) or Estimated Safe and Adequate Daily Dietary Intake (ESADDI) is listed. Major minerals are those with an RDA or ESADDI greater than 100 milligrams, whereas trace minerals have an RDA or ESADDI less than 100 milligrams.

Mineral supplements in various forms have been developed for athletes in attempts to improve performance. In some cases these supplements have been designed to restore those minerals lost from the body during exercise, as the loss might impair performance. In other cases attempts have been made to increase the supply of minerals in the body beyond normal levels in order to improve physiological functioning. The research findings for several minerals will be discussed shortly. Some minerals have been used in combination forms, such as sodium bicarbonate and various phosphate salts; these compounds will be covered in the chapter dealing with physiological ergogenic aids.

TABLE 3.7
**POSSIBLE ROLES OF MINERALS
IMPORTANT DURING EXERCISE**

MINERAL	U.S. RDA OR ESADDI	POSSIBLE ROLE
Calcium	1000 mg	Muscle contraction; glycogen breakdown
Phosphorus	1000 mg	Formation of ATP and CP; release of oxygen from RBC
Magnesium	400 mg	Muscle contraction; glucose metabolism in the muscle cell
Iron	18 mg	Oxygen transport by RBC; oxygen utilization in the muscle cell
Zinc	15 mg	Energy production within muscle cell
Copper	2 mg	Oxygen transport and utilization; close work with iron
Sodium	1100 to 3300 mg	Nerve impulse transmission; muscle contraction; water balance
Potassium	1875 to 5625 mg	Nerve impulse transmission; muscle contraction; glycogen storage

Research Findings

Research studies have shown that minerals may be lost from the body during exercise. One route is through the sweat, which may contain sodium, chloride, and potassium, as well as small amounts of calcium, magnesium, iron, zinc, chromium, and other trace minerals. Another route is the urine, which may contain small amounts of iron, chromium, and copper, among others.

A mineral deficiency *can* have a negative impact upon physical performance, but such a deficiency is rare in athletes. There are occasional case reports in the medical literature of athletes suffering muscle cramps from a deficiency of magnesium, sodium, or potassium, but such cases appear to be uncommon. Most of the research, even in studies where distance runners averaged about 17 miles per day in the heat with copious sweat losses, suggests that if the athlete consumes a balanced diet and returns fluid losses back to normal, mineral balance will be maintained.

Most of the research with supplements has focused on sodium, chloride, and potassium, the major electrolytes found in sweat, and on iron.

Electrolytes and Sports Performance.   During exercise in a warm or hot environment, sweat is evaporated from your skin to help cool your body. Sweat consists primarily of water, with small amounts of sodium, chloride, and potassium. The concentration of these electrolytes in sweat is actually less than their concentration in the body fluids from which sweat is derived; consequently, the concentration of these electrolytes in the blood and body fluids actually increases during exercise. Thus, in most exercise tasks performed in the heat, even in distances up to a marathon run, replacement of these electrolytes is not necessary during the event. Since these electrolytes are extremely important for several vital physiological processes, such as proper functioning of your heart, the body has several very effective mechanisms to prevent excess losses and will restore normal levels on a daily basis.

However, in very prolonged exercise tasks, such as ultramarathon running and Ironman-type triathlons that last more than 6 or 7 hours, electrolyte supplements may be recommended. Several medical reports have revealed that the consumption of only water during ultradistance competition results in a dilution of the sodium content in the body and elicits neurological complications that lead to seizures and the need for hospitilization. This condition of a low level of sodium in the blood is called *hyponatremia* (natrium is Latin for sodium). It is also known as *water intoxication*.

Iron and Sports Performance.   The mineral of most concern to the athlete, especially the endurance athlete, is iron. Iron is a component of *hemoglobin* in the RBC, *myoglobin* in the muscle cell, and some of the oxidative enzymes within the mitochondria (see Figure 3.7). Hemoglobin and myoglobin are carriers of iron. An iron deficiency can impair oxygen transport to the muscles if the hemoglobin level is below normal, and it can impair energy production within the muscle cell if myoglobin and oxidative enzymes are below normal.

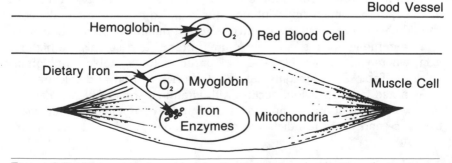

Figure 3.7   Dietary iron is needed for the transport and utilization of oxygen.

Epidemiological research conducted relative to the iron status of athletes has revealed three conditions. Most male and female athletes have normal hemoglobin levels and normal body iron stores. Some male endurance athletes, some female athletes, and many female endurance athletes have normal hemoglobin levels but low body iron stores—a condition known as *iron deficiency without anemia*. A small number of female athletes, particularly distance runners, have both subnormal hemoglobin levels and subnormal body iron stores—a condition known as *iron-deficiency anemia*.

Iron supplements have been used as a means to improve performance in all three conditions. As might be expected, the remediation of iron-deficiency anemia with the return to normal hemoglobin levels through iron supplementation helped to return performance to normal. On the other hand, iron supplementation to athletes with normal hemoglobin levels and iron status had no influence upon endurance performance. The results of research with subjects who have iron deficiency without anemia are contradictory. Most of the research shows that maximal oxygen uptake is not improved, but oxidative processes in the muscle cell may be improved, with a resulting increase in endurance performance. For example, one recent well-designed study with female high school cross-country runners who had iron deficiency without anemia showed that those who had received an iron supplement significantly improved their running time on a treadmill. The other runners showed no improvement.

Recommendations

Minerals in Food.   The general recommendation in order to obtain adequate mineral nutrition is comparable to that for sound vitamin nutrition: Eat a wide variety of foods. You should particularly stress foods rich in iron. Although not discussed above, female athletes should include foods rich in calcium in their diets, for some research suggests that women athletes run a greater risk of stress fractures when they consume lower amounts of calcium. Iron and calcium are two of the key nutrients in the diet. In essence, if you obtain sufficient amounts of these two key minerals, you should obtain an adequate amount of all other minerals you need. In general, lean meats, beans, and whole-grain breads and cereals are high in iron, whereas dairy products and dark green leafy vegetables are high in calcium. Table 3.8 highlights natural foods rich in iron and calcium.

As noted in the previous section with vitamins, some athletes may be on low-calorie diets in attempts to lose weight for competition; others may be concerned that their diets are not providing an adequate supply of

---

TABLE 3.8
FOODS RICH IN IRON AND CALCIUM

IRON	CALCIUM
Meat, fish, and poultry	All dairy products
Liver	Milk, cheese, ice cream, yogurt
Shellfish, especially oysters	Egg yolk
Dried peas and beans	Dried peas and beans
Dark green, leafy vegetables	Dark green, leafy vegetables
Whole-grain products	Cauliflower
Dried apricots, raisins	

---

nutrients. Moreover, many distance runners, particularly females, may be risking iron deficiency due to iron losses in the sweat and urine and an inadequate dietary intake of iron. For example, many athletes today are abstaining from red meat, a good source of iron. In such cases, mineral supplementation may be recommended.

For athletes concerned about nutritional status, the best solution is to consult a nutritionist or a nutritionally oriented physician for a blood and dietary analysis. Unfortunately, most athletes do not take this step; instead they buy nutrient supplements at the local drug store for self-administration. It is important to stress that a mineral supplement should contain only the RDA. Most commercial one-a-day vitamin-mineral supplements are designed to contain the RDA and consequently are safe for most individuals.

Legal, Ethical, and Medical Considerations. At present, mineral supplements are considered legal by sport-governing bodies, so there are no legal or ethical problems. However, megadoses of minerals may cause a variety of health problems. For example, in susceptible individuals excessive amounts of magnesium can cause diarrhea; excess calcium can contribute to the development of kidney stones and abnormal heart rhythms. Potassium supplements can disturb heart function, and excess iron can lead to liver damage. Large single doses of iron can even be fatal.

Water

Theoretical Basis

Water is your most critical nutrient. Your body is approximately 60 percent water, and water is the environment within which all of your other nutrients function. Dehydration, or the loss of body water, can disturb cardiovascular function, cell metabolism, and temperature regulation. Thus, your body has developed several very effective systems to maintain normal body water levels. In essence, the sensation of thirst stimulates you to drink fluids while hormones and other mechanisms regulate the excretion of fluids by your kidneys. Under normal environmental conditions, the sedentary individual consumes and excretes the equivalent of about 2 liters of fluids per day.

Of importance to the athlete is the role that water may play in temperature control and the prevention of dehydration during exercise. As noted previously, exercise increases metabolic heat production. In order to maintain the body temperature in the normal range, this excess heat production must be dissipated. During prolonged exercise in a warm environment, the only effective means to dissipate the heat is through the evaporation of sweat, which is primarily derived from the body water supplies. Thus, unless water is adequately supplied during exercise, excessive dehydration or increases in body temperature may impair performance. In severe cases, temperature regulation may be lost, leading to heatstroke and possibly fatal consequences.

Research Findings

Dehydration and Sports Performance.   Literally thousands of research studies have been conducted to investigate the effect of dehydration and fluid-replenishment techniques on body temperature regulation and physical performance. Many of the earlier studies were done from a military perspective of work performance, but more recent research has focused upon the athlete.

In general, *dehydration leading to body weight losses of only 2 percent may lead to decreases in aerobic endurance capacity*. The greater the fluid loss, the more performance suffers. Although the precise physiological mechanisms through which dehydration impairs aerobic performance are not known, the adverse effects are believed due to inadequate cardiovascular adjustments or to temperature control. For a 150-pound runner, a loss of 3 pounds represents a 2 percent dehydration. In a hot environment, such a loss can occur in less than 30 minutes.

Rehydration and Hyperhydration.   Two techniques have been used successfully to help prevent the adverse effects of dehydration upon aerobic endurance exercise in warm environments. *Rehydration* involves the consumption of fluids during the exercise bout itself, whereas *hyperhydration* involves the intake of fluids prior to exercise. Of the two, rehydration is the most effective means of preventing the adverse effects of dehydration during exercise. However, when compared to conditions in which no fluid is ingested, both techniques have been reported to delay the onset of dehydration, to help maintain cardiovascular function, and to reduce the magnitude of the rise in body temperature during prolonged aerobic exercise in the heat.

Recommendations

If you plan to exercise under warm environmental conditions, both rehydration and hyperhydration techniques are highly recommended. Fluid replacement guidelines recommended for runners may serve as a useful guide.

To hyperhydrate, consume about 1 pint (16 ounces) of cold fluid about 20 to 30 minutes prior to exercise or competition. This should allow enough time for the fluid to evacuate the stomach and yet not trigger a diuretic effect.

To rehydrate, consume about 4 to 8 ounces of cold fluid every 10 to 15 minutes during exercise. Adjust the volume to your individual needs. In prolonged exercise bouts it is important to consume fluids early, for if you wait until you are thirsty you are already in a state of dehydration.

If your exercise task is less than 90 minutes, cold water is the best replacement fluid. In more prolonged exercise, where additional carbohydrates may be beneficial, you may wish to consume some of the carbohydrate solutions discussed earlier in this chapter. Recent research involving rehydration with 5 to 7 percent glucose or glucose-polymer solutions has shown them to be as effective as water in deterring the adverse effects of dehydration during exercise in the heat. In very prolonged exercise tasks, such as ultramarathons and Ironman-type triathlons, the fluid should contain electrolytes, particularly sodium. Small concentrations, like those found in the common commercial products such as Gatorade, appear to be adequate. The consumption of electrolytes may help to prevent hyponatremia, discussed previously.

Legal, Ethical, and Medical Considerations.   There appear to be no legal or medical problems regarding fluid intake prior to or during athletic competition. However, some prolonged endurance events, such as major competitive triathlons, may bar participants from receiving any aid, including fluids, from support teams along the route. In such cases, fluid intake may be, and has been, grounds for disqualification if it has not been obtained at an official aid station.

It should also be noted that even though rehydration and hyperhydration techniques may be beneficial during exercise in the heat, they cannot totally prevent the effects of dehydration and rises in body temperature. Aerobic endurance exercise in the heat will not be as efficient as exercise in a cooler environment. You should expect some slight deterioration in your normal performance.

Ergogenic Foods

Over the years, athletes have used a variety of special foods or food supplements in attempts to improve performance. Honey, gelatin, wheat-germ oil, spirulina, lecithin, ginseng, and others have been advocated in the popular literature for athletes. The available scientific research with these substances has found them to be ineffective ergogenic aids. Nevertheless, manufacturers of supplements for athletes continue to produce new products, and even to recycle old ones, in search of that magical ingredient. Three products recently advertised for athletes are octacosanol, bee pollen, and vitamin B_{15}.

Theoretical Basis

Octacosanol.   Octacosanol, as found in products such as Octacol 4, is a revival of wheat-germ oil, a popular ergogenic aid advertised as the wonder fuel for athletes about 30 years ago. Octacosanol, a white alcohol, was theorized to be the active ingredient in wheat-germ oil. Advertisements suggested it would increase energy and stamina, presumably by increasing oxygen consumption and glycogen metabolism in the muscle.

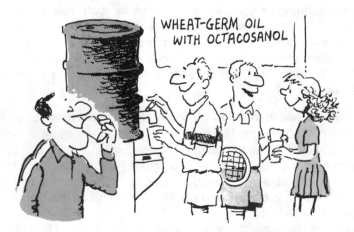

"I think I'm about a quart low."

Bee Pollen.   Bee pollen, analyzed chemically, is a mixture of various vitamins, minerals, amino acids, and other organic compounds. It appears to be a vitamin-mineral supplement. Advertisements have touted its value for helping athletes to recover faster between workouts, thus improving training and competitive performance.

Vitamin B_{15}.   Vitamin B_{15} is actually not a vitamin in the true sense of the term, for there is no known function for it in human nutrition. Chemical analyses of vitamin B_{15} supplements purchased in health food stores have revealed a variety of different components, but the most usual preparation contains a substance known as *calcium pangamate*. Calcium pangamate is a mixture of *calcium gluconate* and *dimethylglycine*, a derived amino acid. Based upon Russian research with rats, these substances are theorized to improve oxidative energy systems in the muscle cells.

Research Findings

A considerable number of earlier studies have been conducted with wheat-germ oil, which contains octacosanol, whereas the research with bee pollen and vitamin B_{15} is more recent.

Octacosanol.   No research has been uncovered to support the contention that octacosanol will improve glycogen metabolism, oxygen consumption, or, for that matter, any other physiological function that would improve physical performance. A careful analysis of over 35 studies with wheat-germ oil, containing octacosanol, led to the conclusion that it was not an effective aid to performance. The Federal Trade Commission recently used this analysis as the basis for banning misleading advertising of improved athletic performance by one manufacturer of wheat-germ oil.

Bee Pollen.   The research findings used by the advertisers of bee pollen to support its effectiveness were derived from a single study, a poorly controlled field study with track athletes. Although this study was never reported in a scientific journal, materials published by the manufacturer claimed improved recovery time in athletes during a track workout. No research has been uncovered to show exactly how bee pollen is supposed to improve performance. In fact, over six well-designed studies have shown that bee pollen will not improve maximal oxygen uptake, other physiological responses to exercise, or various blood characteristics important to performance. The theory of faster recovery times was tested in our laboratory on athletes given various doses of bee pollen. We found bee pollen to be ineffective with highly trained runners.

Vitamin B_{15}.   As noted above, most of the research in support of vitamin B_{15} as an effective supplement for human athletes has been extrapolated from research with rats, and the results of most of this research are question-able. Four recent well-designed studies with humans have revealed that B_{15} supplements have no effect on cardiovascular or metabolic responses to exercise, maximal oxygen uptake, or maximal endurance performance.

Recommendations

As is obvious from the summarization of the research findings, octacosanol, bee pollen, and vitamin B_{15} have little theoretical or experimental research support as means of improving athletic performance. You are advised to save your money and avoid these products.

Legal, Ethical, and Medical Considerations.   Although these compounds appear to be legal and are not banned by sport-governing bodies, there may be some health risks involved with taking them. Several cases of al-lergies to bee pollen ingestion have been reported in the medical litera-ture. Also, recent chemical analyses of vitamin B_{15} compounds have revealed the presence of several ingredients known to be mutagenic to humans.

Selected Readings

Books

Clark, N. (1981). *The athlete's kitchen*. Cambridge: CBI Publishing.
National Association for Sport and Physical Education. (1984). *Nutrition for sport success*. Reston, VA: American Alliance for Health, Physi-cal Education, Recreation and Dance.
Williams, M. (1985). *Nutritional aspects of human physical and athletic performance*. Springfield, IL: Charles C. Thomas.
Williams, M. (1988). *Nutrition for fitness and sport*. Dubuque: Brown.

Reviews

American Dietetic Association. (1980). Nutrition and physical fitness. *Journal of the American Dietetic Association, **76**,* 437-443.
Belko, A. (1987). Vitamins and exercise: An update. *Medicine and Science in Sports and Exercise, **19**,* S191-S196.
Blom, P., Costill, D., & Vollestad, N. (1987). Exhaustive running: In-appropriate as a stimulus of muscle glycogen supercompensation. *Medicine and Science in Sports and Exercise, **19**,* 398-403.

Brotherhood, J. (1984). Nutrition and sports performance. *Sports Medicine,* **1**, 350-389.

Bruce, A., Ekblom, B., & Nilsson, I. (1985). The effect of vitamin and mineral supplements and health foods on physical endurance and performance. *Proceedings of the Nutrition Society,* **44**, 283-295.

Clement, D., & Sawchuck, L. (1984). Iron status and sports performance. *Sports Medicine,* **1**, 65-74.

Conlee, R. (1987). Muscle glycogen and exercise endurance: A twenty-year perspective. *Exercise and Sport Science Reviews,* **15**, 1-28.

Costill, D., & Miller, J. (1980). Nutrition for endurance sport: Carbohydrate and fluid balance. *International Journal of Sports Medicine,* **1**, 2-14.

Gisolfi, C. (1986). Impact of limited fluid intake on performance. In Committee on Military Nutrition (Eds.), *Predicting decrements in military performance due to inadequate nutrition* (pp. 17-28). Washington, DC: National Academy Press.

Haymes, E. (1987). Nutritional concerns: Need for iron. *Medicine and Science in Sports and Exercise,* **19**, S197-S200.

Lemon, P. (1987). Protein and exercise: Update 1987. *Medicine and Science in Sports and Exercise,* **19**, S179-S190.

Lemon, P., Yarasheski, K., & Dolny, D. (1984). The importance of protein for athletes. *Sports Medicine,* **1**, 474-484.

Sherman, W. (1987). Carbohydrate, muscle glycogen, and improved performance. *The Physician and Sportsmedicine,* **15**(2), 157-164.

Sherman, W., & Costill, D. (1984). The marathon: Dietary manipulation to optimize performance. *American Journal of Sports Medicine,* **12**, 44-51.

Slavin, J., Landers, G., & Engstrom, M. (1988). Amino acid supplements: Beneficial or risky? *The Physician and Sportsmedicine,* **16**(3), 221-224.

Van der Beek, E. (1985). Vitamins and endurance training: Food for running and faddish claims. *Sports Medicine,* **2**, 175-197.

Williams, C. (1985). Nutritional aspects of exercise-induced fatigue. *Proceedings of the Nutrition Society,* **44**, 245-256.

Williams, M. (1981). Vitamin, iron and calcium supplementation: Effect on human physical performance. In W. Haskell, J. Scala, & J. Whittam (Eds.), *Nutrition and athletic performance* (pp. 106-153). Palo Alto: Bull Publishing.

Williams, M. (1986). Minerals and physical performance. In Committee on Military Nutrition (Eds.), *Predicting decrements in military performance due to inadequate nutrition* (pp. 163-187). Washington, DC: National Academy Press.

Wilmore, J., & Freund, B. (1986). Nutritional enhancement of athletic performance. *Current Concepts in Nutrition,* **15**, 67-97.

Young, V. (1986). Protein and amino acid metabolism in relation to physical exercise. *Current Concepts in Nutrition,* **15**, 9-32.

Chapter 4

Pharmacological
Ergogenic Aids

THE ERGOGENIC AIDS THAT HAVE RAISED the most concern among athletic-governing bodies are the pharmacological agents, or drugs. *Doping*, or the use of drugs by athletes in attempts to improve performance, has persisted for nearly a century, but it was not until after World War II that doping became rampant among athletes involved in international competition and professional sports. Doping eventually filtered down to college sports, and today appears to pervade sports at even the high school level.

Although doping in sports was a growing concern, drug use was not regulated until the death of a cyclist in the 1960 Olympic Games in Rome triggered the formation of the Medical Commission of the International Olympic Committee (IOC) and the initiation of anti-doping legislation for Olympic competition. The legislation developed by the IOC serves as a guideline for other athletic-governing bodies, such as the International Amateur Cycling Federation, The Athletics Congress (TAC), and the National Collegiate Athletic Association (NCAA). The general definition of doping as developed by the IOC is as follows:

> Doping is the administration of or the use by a competing athlete of any substance foreign to the body or of any physiological substance taken in abnormal quantity or by an abnormal route of entry into the body, with the intention of increasing in an artificial and unfair manner his performance in competition. When necessity demands medical treatment with any substance which because of its nature, dosage, or application is able to boost the athlete's performance in competition in an artifical and unfair manner, this is to be regarded as doping. (Clarke, 1972, p. 28)

The major purpose of this general rule was to discourage the use of drugs by athletes, and in this regard the IOC lists several pages of specific drugs banned in athletic competition. There is no need to list these specific drugs, for terms such as phendimetrazine, etafedreine, bemigride, and fluoxymesterone may not be very meaningful to you. However, the IOC does group these specific drugs into several distinct categories, such as stimulants, depressants, diuretics, and anabolic steroids, and this categorization will serve as the basis for the discussion in this chapter. An expanded list of drugs banned by the IOC and/or the NCAA may be found in the appendix.

Before we begin our discussion of some of the more obvious and commonly used drugs used to improve performance in sports, it is important to point out that all of the agents discussed in this chapter, with some exceptions and limitations that shall be noted, are banned for use by most athletic-governing bodies and are thus illegal for athletes to use (see appendix).

In order to enforce anti-doping legislation, a highly technical and effective drug-testing system is available to most athletic-governing bodies. However, like many athletes, you may take drugs for a variety of medicinal purposes, such as a headache, a stuffed nose, a cold, or to heal an injury. Unfortunately, many over-the-counter medications that you may be able to purchase without a prescription for such conditions may contain drugs that are banned for athletic competition. Several examples are Sudafed, Dristan, Sinex, and Nyquil. If you will be competing in any athletic event involving drug testing, such as a TAC-sponsored road race or NCAA contest, it would be advisable to check with the athletic-governing body about the legality of any medications you are taking.

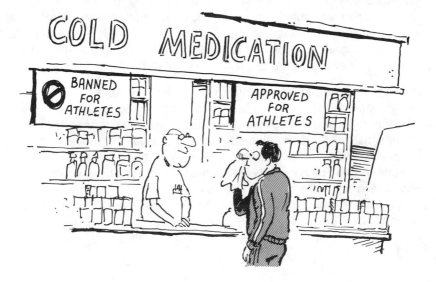

Stimulants

Theoretical Basis

By medical definition stimulants are agents that help to increase functional ability, so any agent that might be able to improve functions important to athletic success may be an effective ergogenic aid. Examples of stimulants are *caffeine*, *amphetamines*, *ephedrine* (in nasal decongestants), *nicotine*, and *cocaine*. As a matter of fact, stimulants have been one of the most popular doping agents used in modern athletics. Their use and abuse in professional baseball and football have been well documented. As mentioned previously, the use of amphetamines during the 1960 Olympic Games and a resultant fatality provided the stimulus for the development of the IOC antidoping rules. The current list of drugs banned by the IOC contains over 40 different stimulants (see appendix).

Use of Stimulants. Most of us consume stimulant drugs in one form or another almost daily. The most common stimulant available to us is, of course, *caffeine*, which is found in such beverages and foods as coffee, cocoa, tea, chocolate, and cola sodas. Caffeine is also found in aspirin, whereas many other over-the-counter preparations that we may take contain various stimulant drugs on the IOC doping list. For example, many nasal decongestants contain *ephedrine*, a stimulant that resulted in the loss of a gold medal when inadvertently used by an American swimmer in the 1972 Olympic games.

A wide variety of stimulant drugs has been developed by medical researchers. Many of these drugs are designed to exert only very specific local effects. For example, *digitalis* is a cardiac stimulant designed to increase the contractile force of the heart, and thus is an important medication for some cardiac patients. On the other hand, many stimulant drugs exert widespread psychological and physiological effects throughout the body; it is this type of stimulant drug that has been of interest to athletes as a means of improving performance.

Historically, *amphetamines* have been the most widely used stimulant among athletes at all levels of competition. More recently, caffeine has become popular among many athletes, particularly endurance runners and cyclists. Although there may be some small differences in the psychological and physiological effects that various stimulants may exert in the body, there are many similarities regarding their possible effects on functions that are important during competition in sport.

Psychological Effects. Psychologically, such stimulants as amphetamines and caffeine may increase excitability, arousal, attention, concentration, motivation, and self-confidence, while concomitantly removing psychological inhibitions. In other words, psychological energy is increased. It is obvious that this psychological stimulation could be important to athletes in a variety of sports if it would add to the normal stimulation elicited by athletic competition itself. For example, greater concentration in a tennis player might result in a faster reaction to a return. On the other hand, excessive excitability resulting in muscle tremor and unsteadiness may be deleterious to some athletic performances, such as archery and riflery.

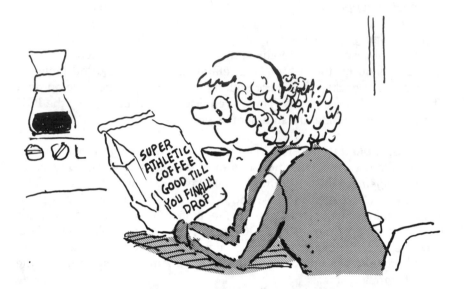

Physiological Effects.   Physiologically, stimulants have been used by athletes because they produce physiological responses in the body comparable to that of *epinephrine*, also called *adrenalin*, which is a natural hormone secreted by the adrenal gland. During exercise, your sympathetic nervous system activates the adrenal gland, which releases epinephrine into the blood for delivery to all tissues. Many stimulant drugs mimic this natural action of the sympathetic nervous system and thus are called *sympathomimetic* drugs. The resulting physiological responses that could be important for energy production during exercise include facilitation of contractile processes in the muscle, increased size of the bronchi delivering air to the lungs, increased amount of blood pumped by the heart, increased blood flow to the muscle, and increased availability of glucose and free fatty acids (FFA) in the blood to serve as energy sources. Many of these changes could be theorized to benefit the oxygen energy system and, thereby, aerobic endurance. One current popular theory suggests that the increased levels of blood FFA will increase the use of fat as an energy source in the muscle, thereby improving performance by sparing muscle glycogen for use during the latter stages of a prolonged endurance event.

In summary, stimulants are theorized to improve athletic performance, either through psychological or physiological mechanisms, and to increase energy production, but only if they can augment the natural psychological and physiological effects induced by the secretion of natural hormones in the body during athletic competition. On the other hand, as we shall see, there may be some potential adverse effects of these agents upon physical performance.

Research Findings

Most of the research concerning stimulants and physical performance has focused upon amphetamines and caffeine, although some data are available with stimulants found in asthmatic medications, nicotine in cigarettes and smokeless tobacco, and cocaine.

Physiological and Performance Effects. Although research does show that most of these stimulants may elicit physiological responses in the body at rest that may have important implications for exercise, such as increased blood flow from the heart, the vast majority of the research available suggests that none of these stimulants appears to benefit physiological functioning during exercise. Heart rate, blood flow, lung ventilation, and oxygen uptake are not improved by stimulant drugs during maximal exercise. Apparently the natural release of epinephrine and other stimulants in the body during exercise override the effects of stimulant drugs and no additional physiological benefits occur.

Even though physiological functions during exercise do not appear to be enhanced by stimulants, evidence suggests that certain stimulants may improve actual physical performance itself, most likely through psychological mechanisms. Studies with strong stimulants, such as amphetamines, have reported improved reaction time in fatigued subjects as well as increases in strength and power in rested subjects. Amphetamines have also been shown to improve performance in tests of local muscular endurance to fatigue, not by directly improving energy production in the muscle but by increasing the psychological tolerance to pain, as evidenced by larger levels of lactic acid in the blood. Caffeine is a weaker stimulant than amphetamines, and beneficial effects of caffeine on fitness components, such as reaction time, strength, power, and local muscular endurance, are not as well supported by the available research.

One of the more consistent, although not universal, research findings with stimulants is an improvement in aerobic endurance performance. A number of studies with amphetamines or caffeine have documented improved endurance capacity, usually measured by exercise tests to exhaustion, about 50 to 120 minutes on a bicycle ergometer or treadmill. With caffeine, the dosage may be important. In one recent study endurance performance was significantly improved when the dosage was 15 milligrams per kilogram of body weight, but performance was not affected with only 10 milligrams per kilogram. It should be noted that even a dose of 10 milligrams per kilogram of body weight is beyond the permissible level specified by the IOC doping rule.

In attempts to determine why these stimulants improve aerobic endurance, much of the recent research along these lines has looked at the role of caffeine as a means to spare muscle glycogen by increasing the utilization of FFA as an energy source during exercise (see Figure 3.4 in the preceding chapter). Although some research data do suggest that caffeine may facilitate the use of fats stored in the muscle as an energy source during exercise, its ability to spare muscle glycogen stores is not well documented. In essence, no physiological factor has been identified as the means of improving performance. Thus, most investigators in this area suggest that the improved endurance may be due to improved psychological functioning that leads to greater work output or increased tolerance to fatigue. In support of this contention, one study revealed that caffeine elicited a decreased level of psychological stress during a 90-minute treadmill run when compared to a trial with a placebo.

Nicotine and Marijuana.   Another readily available stimulant is nicotine, found in cigarettes and *smokeless tobacco*. Some athletes have been known to smoke a cigarette prior to an event or chew tobacco during competition for the stimulating effect. However, there is little evidence available to support the effectiveness of either practice. Research with smoking has actually shown an increased resistance to breathing and decreases in maximal oxygen uptake and endurance performance, which may be partially attributed to other factors in cigarette smoke besides nicotine. The limited research available regarding the effects of smokeless tobacco on athletic performance suggests tobacco has no beneficial effects upon reaction time, movement time, or total response time, and thus does not appear to be an effective ergogenic aid for those athletes who use it the most, baseball players.

Marijuana smoking also induces some stimulant effects. Research has shown that marijuana may cause increased secretion of epinephrine in the body, resulting in an increased heart rate and bronchial dilation. However, several well-controlled studies have shown that although marijuana smoking exerts little effect on physiological measurements during exercise, such as maximal oxygen uptake, endurance performance is nevertheless impaired. Furthermore, other research has shown that fine motor tasks may also be impaired following marijuana smoking.

In summary, some laboratory and field research has supported the role of several stimulants as a means of improving physical performance. The

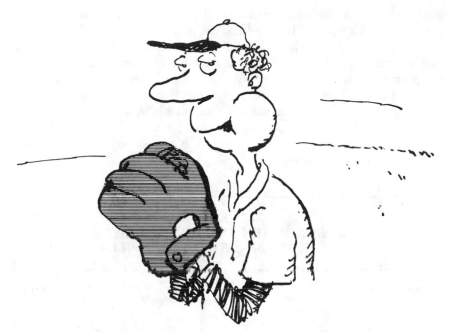

Some people think that nicotine is an ergogenic aid.

evidence may possibly be extrapolated to actual athletic competition. However, it is possible that the psychological environment normally associated with athletic competition will itself provide an adequate natural stimulant effect and that additional stimulants are not helpful.

Recommendations

Amphetamines.   Strong stimulants such as amphetamines are not recommended because of possible medical complications. Amphetamines appear to disturb normal temperature regulation, which may lead to serious heat illness, such as heatstroke. They increase diuresis and body water losses; increase the basal metabolic rate and body temperature; restrict blood flow to the skin, which hinders heat loss; interfere with the role of the hypothalamus in temperature control; and help to mask fatigue, allowing the athlete to push beyond normal limits. All of these factors can contribute in raising the body temperature to dangerous levels. Furthermore, because they increase muscular tremor and anxiety levels, amphetamines may actually lead to deterioration in sports where fine motor control is essential. Finally, in large doses amphetamines may be fatal.

Caffeine.   Because caffeine is an ingredient in beverages and foods commonly consumed by athletes, its use is permitted by the IOC, but only in limited amounts. The IOC permits an upper limit of 15 micrograms per milliliter of urine tested. This would be the equivalent of 15 milligrams per liter of water in the body of the athlete. A male athlete who weighs 154 pounds, or 70 kilograms, and whose body composition contains 60 percent water will have about 42 liters of water in his body, as .60 × 70 = 42, and a kilogram of water is one liter. If you multiply 15 milligrams by 42 liters, you will find that this athlete may consume about 630 milligrams of caffeine to reach the legal limit. As noted in Table 4.1, 630 milligrams would be equivalent to 5 or 6 cups of coffee. (For equivalent doses of other beverages and pills, see Table 4.1.)

TABLE 4.1
**APPROXIMATE CAFFEINE CONTENT
IN COMMON BEVERAGES AND PILLS**

Brewed coffee, cup	100 to 125 mg
Decaffeinated coffee, cup	3 to 5 mg
Medium-brewed tea, cup	50 to 70 mg
Cocoa, cup	10 to 15 mg
Cola-type soda, glass	45 to 65 mg
Aspirin tablet	15 to 35 mg
No-Doz tablet	100 mg

Nevertheless, depending upon the individual, a range of 100 to 300 milligrams of caffeine is considered a therapeutic dose. Thus, several cups of brewed coffee or two No-Doz tablets could provide a therapeutic dose and yet still be legal according to IOC doping standards. For athletes who feel they benefit from caffeine, about 5 milligrams per kilogram of body weight may be a recommended legal dose. Simply determine your weight in kilograms by dividing your weight in pounds by 2.2, then multiply the result by 5. Thus, a recommended dose for a 132-pound athlete (60 kilograms) would be 300 milligrams (5 × 60). Recommended doses for lighter and heavier athletes would be lower and higher, respectively. Such doses meet the level for a stimulant effect and are still legal under IOC guidelines. However, it should be noted that not all research has supported the effectiveness of caffeine as a means of improving sport performance.

Many endurance athletes consume caffeine in the belief that the glycogen-sparing theory works. If so, they may want to abstain from caffeine for several days prior to competition. Most individuals develop a tolerance to caffeine and thus need larger doses to experience an effect. However, recent research has shown that abstaining from caffeine for 4 days will diminish this tolerance somewhat, allowing caffeine ingestion to produce a more potent effect, such as a greater rise in blood FFA.

On the other hand, research has also shown that a high-carbohydrate diet and carbohydrate intake prior to competition will blunt the effect of the caffeine. The high-carbohydrate diet may stimulate insulin release, which will inhibit the release of FFA. Since carbohydrate loading and carbohydrate intake appear to be more effective in benefiting endurance performance, the normal dietary practices undertaken by most endurance athletes prior to competition may negate any physiological benefits from caffeine.

Furthermore, caffeine is not without any potential adverse side effects for the endurance athlete. Caffeine is a diuretic; it also increases the basal metabolic rate and heat production. Both of these physiological effects could contribute to inadequate temperature regulation during exercise in warm environmental conditions.

If you regularly consume products containing caffeine and experience few problems, you may wish to experiment with caffeine as an ergogenic aid. Abstain for a few days and consume about two cups of coffee before a long training run or other endurance task. Perform these endurance tasks periodically both with and without the caffeine and judge for yourself if caffeine works for you. You may want to note the time it takes you to do the task and how difficult it was on a scale of 1 to 10. To make it a more valid case study, have a friend prepare for you either regular or decaffeinated coffee and not let you know which you have consumed until after you have compared several exercise trials with coffee, decaffeinated coffee, and no coffee. In this way you can eliminate the placebo effect.

Finally, caffeine is a drug, and individuals respond differently to drugs. In many of the studies, some subjects experienced adverse reactions, particularly subjects who normally did not consume caffeine, and performance suffered. If you are susceptible to some of the adverse effects of caffeine, such as nervousness and anxiety, then caffeine will most likely be counterproductive for you.

Nicotine and Marijuana.   Because nicotine has not been shown to improve physical performance and marijuana may actually decrease performance, there is little basis to recommend their use. Moreover, the usual means of ingesting these drugs (smoking and smokeless tobacco) may carry serious long-term health risks, including coronary heart disease and various forms of cancer. Interestingly, marijuana is not officially banned by the IOC or USOC, but is banned by the NCAA.

Legal, Ethical, and Medical Considerations.   There are some bona fide medical applications for stimulants. For example, amphetamines have been used to treat certain sleep disorders, whereas ephedrine and other stimulants are common ingredients in medicines for the treatment of asthma, a condition found in a significant number of athletes. However, since these agents are on the IOC doping list, there is no legal basis for recommending their use in sport. In certain cases, however, the IOC may approve certain asthmatic drugs if the condition cannot be controlled by permissible medications. As already noted, several of these stimulants may carry significant health risks and thus also may not be recommended from a medical standpoint.

Depressants

Theoretical Basis

In contrast to stimulants, which are designed to increase physiological functions in the body, depressant drugs are utilized to decrease the functional activity of the central nervous system or specific body systems. In this regard, a wide variety of drugs, such as *alcohol, morphine, tranquilizers,* and *beta-blockers,* may be classified as depressants (see appendix). For example, morphine may depress the entire central nervous system, whereas beta-blockers are primarily designed to affect the cardiovascular system, reducing overexcitability of the heart in cardiac patients or individuals with high blood pressure. Morphine is classified as a true depressant; although beta-blockers are not technically classified as depressants, they do lead to the depression of some body functions.

As with stimulant drugs, different depressants vary in their potency. For example, *aspirin* is a mild analgesic used to depress the sensation of pain, *mild tranquilizers* may induce a state of relaxation, and stronger *narcotics,* such as morphine, may induce unconsciousness. The potency also depends upon the dosage. All of these depressant drugs may fulfill their designated function in medicine with an appropriate dose, but all may be fatal if overdosed.

Use of Depressants.   You may wonder why depressants would be used by athletes, as they actually depress physiological functions. As a matter of fact, the term *doping* at one time had negative connotations in sport. Depressant drugs were often surreptitiously given to opponents, such as boxers, racehorses, or greyhounds, in order to impair their performance.

There are several reasons athletes may use depressants in attempts to improve performance. First, some depressants are used to increase the tolerance to pain during exercise or for the paradoxical stimulating effect they achieve by releasing inhibitions and thus allowing an athlete to perform beyond normal limitations. Second, some depressants have been used to increase the self-confidence of the athlete. These effects could benefit athletes in a wide variety of sports where strength, power, and endurance are important.

A third reason for the use of depressants is to reduce anxiety levels and muscle tremor during competition. Such athletes as ballet dancers, figure skaters, ski jumpers, and those in shooting and archery competition may suffer decreases in performance if they are overly excited. In these cases such depressants as tranquilizers, alcohol, and beta-blockers have been utilized in attempts to induce a calming effect. Beta-blockers appear to be popular among shooters and archers, as they are theorized to improve performance in two ways: (a) steadying the arm through reduction of muscle tremors, and (b) slowing the heart rate so the athlete has more time to fire between heartbeats when the body is not moved slightly by the heart contraction.

The IOC has banned most depressants because they may be harmful to injured athletes who still desire to compete. The use of strong pain killers by injured athletes in order to enable them to continue in competition may lead to more severe and possibly permanent injury. Furthermore, many of these drugs are addictive and may lead to serious personal, psychological, and social problems.

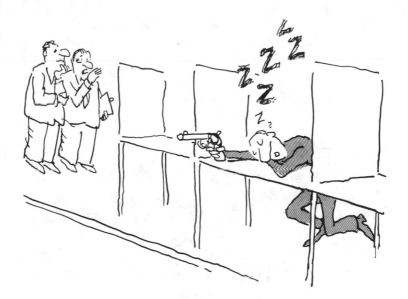

"These depressants really relax my shooters."

Research Findings

Most of the research relative to the effects of depressants on physical perfor-mance has involved the use of mild tranquilizers and alcohol. More re-cently, many studies have focused on the role of beta-blockers. The usual research protocols were designed to evaluate the acute ergogenic effects of the drug by administering a specific dose, waiting for it to take effect, and then testing performance. Many studies with alcohol involved several different dosages. In order to simplify the interpretation of the numerous studies available, we shall divide the analysis into two aspects. We shall look first at the effect of these depressants upon physiological functions and physical performance skills important to most athletes and then look at the research specifically with athletes involved in shooting and archery competition.

Physiological, Psychomotor, and Performance Effects.   In general, alco-hol and mild tranquilizers will impair performance that involves the need for rapid decision making. For example, although the response of each individual following the ingestion of alcohol is unique, some studies have reported that the alcohol content in one drink, such as 12 ounces of beer, may slow reaction time and impair judgment in some subjects. Other im-portant psychomotor abilities such as balance, hand-eye coordination, and arm steadiness may deteriorate with higher dosages. Literally hundreds of studies involving alcohol, and several involving mild tranquilizers, are available to support the fact that athletic performances involving the need to make quick judgments and react to rapidly changing stimuli are adversely affected by the consumption of these drugs.

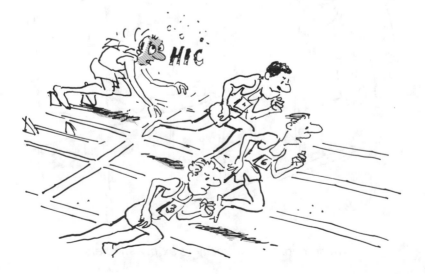

However, one of the most consistent findings with alcohol and mild tranquilizers is the absence during maximal exercise tests of any effect upon physiological functions, such as lung ventilation, heart rate, cardiac output, blood flow, availability of glucose or FFA to the muscle, blood lactate levels, and maximal oxygen uptake. Moreover, actual performances on tests of strength, power, anaerobic endurance, and aerobic endurance have neither improved nor deteriorated with these drugs. It appears that though alcohol or mild tranquilizers will not lead to a decrement in these types of athletic performances, as contrasted to psychomotor skills, neither will performance be improved.

On the other hand, beta-blockers may exert some adverse effects on aerobic endurance performance. Beta-blockers are designed to counteract the actions of several natural stimulants found in the body, namely epinephrine and norepinephrine, and thus may be valuable drugs for the treatment of some heart problems and high blood pressure (see Figure 4.1). Since epinephrine is also an important hormone involved in the body's response to exercise, beta-blockers may block some of these beneficial effects of epinephrine. Indeed, research with highly trained athletes during exercise has shown that beta-blockers will decrease the response of the heart, the blood flow to the muscle, maximal oxygen uptake, and the blood levels of glucose and FFA. These physiological changes were related to a significant decrease in aerobic endurance performance.

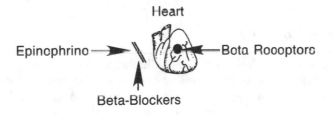

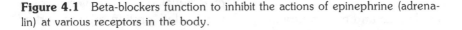

Figure 4.1   Beta-blockers function to inhibit the actions of epinephrine (adrenalin) at various receptors in the body.

Shooting and Archery Performance.   Several studies have investigated the efficacy of depressants on performance in shooting and archery events. An early report noted that both alcohol and tranquilizers improved pistol-shooting accuracy, but the placebo was also effective so no valid conclusions could be made. In a recent well-controlled study with archers, alcohol exerted some contrasting effects. First, small doses of alcohol elicited no effect on strength or endurance. Second, alcohol resulted in slower reaction times and a decrease in hand steadiness—factors that would impair performance. But, third, the use of alcohol also resulted in a smoother release of the arrow, which would improve performance. Unfortunately, no actual performance data were collected. Although athletes in these events are known to use alcohol and tranquilizers for competitive purposes, the available research is not conclusive that such practices are truly beneficial.

In contrast, recent research with beta-blockers supports their value as an effective ergogenic aid for marksmen and markswomen. In a double-blind, placebo study with 33 skilled marksmen, beta-blockers decreased the emotional increases in heart rate and blood pressure often associated with shooting competition, decreased anxiety, and decreased the perceived feelings of tension in the athletes. Pistol-shooting performance improved by over 13 percent, the improvement being attributed to a decrease in muscle tremor and greater steadiness.

In summary, with the exception of the shooting events, it appears obvious that depressants do not benefit athletic performance and may actually hurt it. However, because alcohol is an ingredient in many beverages consumed by athletes on a social basis and beta-blockers may be used by some athletes to control high blood pressure, their use is not banned in most Olympic events. At present, these agents are banned for athletes in the 11 pistol and riflery events and the 2 archery events in Olympic competition as well as in other sports where excess anxiety may interfere with performance, such as figure skating, ski jumping, diving, fencing, gymnastics, and synchronized swimming.

Recommendations

Social Use of Alcohol.   For those athletes who do consume alcohol on a social basis, it appears that one or two drinks the night before competition will not have any deleterious effects on performance the following day. However, excessive consumption may. Visual disturbances have been reported following a night of heavy drinking, so athletes who rely on accurate vision, such as shooters, may be affected adversely. Moreover, alcohol is a diuretic and may contribute to a state of dehydration prior to performance if the athlete does not properly rehydrate. Thus, endurance athletes performing in the heat may be at a disadvantage.

Finally, the consumption of alcohol, usually in the form of beer, is a common practice after many athletic events, particularly road races. Although the water in beer may aid rehydration and the alcohol may produce a state of relaxation, the athlete is more prone to possible adverse effects. The stomach of the athlete is empty and the body dehydrated, so the alcohol is absorbed more readily and is not diluted as much, leading to a rapid rise in the blood alcohol level. As is obvious from highway statistics, operation of an automobile, which involves fine motor control and rapid judgment, under such conditions may be dangerous.

Legal, Ethical, and Medical Considerations.   The research suggests that the only effective application of depressants as ergogenic aids would be in sports where excess anxiety and nervousness could impair performance, such as in shooting events. However, because they are banned by the governing bodies of several sports, their use cannot be recommended. Furthermore, because depressants such as alcohol may deteriorate performance in athletic events requiring rapid judgment and fine motor control, and because beta-blockers may impair aerobic endurance capacity, their use in sports may actually be detrimental.

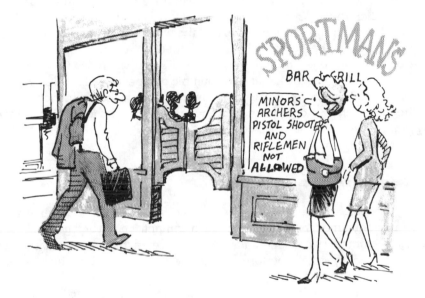

Diuretics

Theoretical Basis

Diuretics represent a class of drugs that increase the secretion of urine. They may either increase the blood flow to the kidneys and hence increase the filtration rate, or they may decrease the absorption of fluid as it passes along the kidney tubules. Diuretics have been popular drugs in the treatment of high blood pressure, but due to adverse side effects their use is on the wane.

One of the reasons athletes have used diuretics is not for a direct ergogenic effect, but rather to avoid detection of the use of illegal pharmacological ergogenic aids. Because of their ability to increase urine production and secretion, some diuretics may also increase the excretion rate of certain banned drugs. Some athletes hope the use of diuretics will help them to excrete the banned drug prior to the urine test that determines drug use.

Athletes in sports such as boxing, wrestling, and judo may use diuretics to lose weight rapidly in order to qualify for a particular weight-class in competition. Gymnasts, jockeys, high jumpers, and athletes in other sports where excess body weight may be a disadvantage may also use diuretics. Diuretics may induce a 3 percent or greater reduction in body weight within a relatively short period of time. For a 160-pound athlete, this would be approximately 5 pounds. If these body water losses do not impair performance, then the wrestler in the lower weight class, the gymnast with less weight to support on the side horse, and the high jumper with a few pounds less to get over the bar may have a competitive advantage.

For these reasons, the IOC has recently added diuretics to the list of drugs banned for use by athletes in Olympic competition. The NCAA and other athletic-governing bodies also ban their use. It should be noted that although alcohol and caffeine have been banned by the IOC for other reasons, they can also act as diuretics.

Research Findings

Body Weight.   Based on the laws of physics, it is logical to assume that a wrestler, gymnast, or high jumper is at a competitive advantage at a lower weight. Although little evidence has been uncovered that documents a direct improvement in athletic performance following the use of diuretics, some recent data suggest beneficial effects.

In general, research with diuretics has shown that they may lead to substantial body water losses, over 3 percent, and not result in any deterioration in strength, power, or local muscular endurance of an anaerobic nature. Thus, in sports characterized by brief, intense effort, performance would seemingly not be compromised by use of diuretic agents and may be benefited. For example, a recent study revealed that the use of a diuretic, or the combination of dieting and a diuretic, to lose weight led to improvement in vertical jumping ability. The effects of body weight on other forms of sports performance will be discussed further in chapter 7.

Aerobic Endurance.   The use of diuretics may lead to a significant deterioration in aerobic endurance performance. Research has shown the dehydration caused by diuretics may produce a decrease in the plasma volume of 8 to 10 percent even though total body weight loss is only

3 percent. This decrease in plasma volume has resulted in impaired cardio-vascular functions during exercise, such as a decrease in the amount of blood pumped per beat. Although research generally has not found a decrease in maximal oxygen uptake with the use of diuretics, endurance performance has suffered. In one of the most interesting research projects, investigators studied running performance in three races of different lengths—1.5, 5, and 10 kilometers—in order to test the effects of diuretic-induced dehydration. Compared to a placebo condition, performance times after using diuretics were about 8 seconds slower in the 1.5-kilometer race, 78 seconds slower in the 5-kilometer, and 157 seconds slower in the 10-kilometer.

Furthermore, research findings presented in the previous chapter relative to the detrimental effects of exercise-induced or thermal-induced dehydration upon exercise performance under warm environmental conditions are applicable to diuretic-induced dehydration.

Recommendations

Legal, Ethical, and Medical Considerations. Because diuretics are banned agents there is no legal or ethical basis to recommend their use by athletes. Although most medical authorities decry the use of various weight loss practices used in some sports, wrestlers and other athletes continue to use them. Most athletes can reach their desired body weight through a proper nutritional program and safe, legal dehydration techniques such as exercise.

As previously noted, the use of diuretics is not recommended in sports involving aerobic endurance because performance will deteriorate.

Diuretic-induced dehydration may also pose some serious health problems to athletes, for athletes will be more susceptible to heat exhaustion or heatstroke while exercising in warm temperatures. Also, besides water, diuretics also excrete electrolytes such as potassium. Thus, the chronic use of diuretics may lead to low levels of body potassium and disturbed neurological functioning, with symptoms ranging from muscular weakness to disturbances of normal heart function, even heart failure.

Anabolic Steroids

Theoretical Basis

Anabolic steroids represent a class of drugs of which use among athletes has reached epidemic proportions. It has been estimated that over one million Americans use anabolic steroids, including many male and female athletes varying in age from the mature professional down to the junior high school student who has not passed through puberty. Since steroids are prescription drugs, a flourishing black market approximating $100 million in yearly sales has developed and appears to be centered around local gyms and health clubs that stress strength training and bodybuilding.

The Testosterone Effect.   Anabolic steroids are popular among athletes because they mimic the effects of the natural male sex hormone, testosterone (see Figure 4.2). Testosterone produces two major effects in the body, *androgenic* and *anabolic*, which are most evident at the onset of puberty in boys. Androgenic changes involve such secondary sex characteristics in the male as facial hair, a deeper voice, and maturation of the sex glands. Anabolic changes include growth and development of many body tissues, the most obvious change at puberty being the rapid increases in muscle mass.

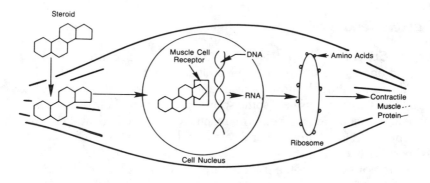

Figure 4.2   Anabolic steroids picked up by receptors in the cell nucleus initiate the process of protein formation in cells such as muscle fibers.

Natural testosterone itself was used over 50 years ago in attempts to improve physical performance by increasing anabolism. Unfortunately, natural testosterone also causes its normal androgenic effects, which may be undesirable to some. Thus, chemists rearranged the structure of the testosterone molecule in order to maximize the anabolic effects and minimize the androgenic effects. Nevertheless, all anabolic steroids do produce some androgenic effects. Anabolic steroids are available for oral consumption or injection. A few of the more popular anabolic steroids are listed in Table 4.2.

Anabolic steroids have a bona fide role in medicine. They may be used effectively for the treatment of certain forms of anemia and osteoporosis and for the prevention of muscle wasting in certain diseases. They were used quite extensively following World War II to help restore body tissues

TABLE 4.2
**TRADE AND GENERIC NAMES OF THE MOST COMMONLY
USED ANABOLIC STEROIDS IN THE UNITED STATES**

ORAL COMPOUNDS

Anadrol (oxymetholone)

Anavar (oxandrolone)

Dianabol (methandienone)

Maxibolin (ethylestrenol)

Winstrol (stanozolol)

INJECTABLE COMPOUNDS

Deca-durabolin (nandrolone decanoate)

Depo-testosterone (testosterone cypionate)

Durabolin (nandrolone phenylpropionate)

Primobolan-depot (methenolone enanthate)

in victims of enforced starvation. However, their ability to increase muscle mass in normal individuals was quickly recognized, and their application to sport began in earnest in the early 1950s. By the 1960s physicians were prescribing them for use by athletes, and one pharmaceutical company even advertised their value to increase muscle mass. As has been noted, they remain among the most popular drugs used by athletes today.

Physiological and Psychological Effects.   Athletes may take anabolic steroids for a variety of reasons, some physiological and some psychological. However, in contrast to the stimulants and depressants, they do not take steroids on the day of competition for the acute effect, but rather use them as an adjunct to their training for months prior to the competition. Steroids are designed to provide an effect above and beyond the normal effects of training.

As is probably obvious by now, the primary physiological purpose for using anabolic steroids is to increase muscle mass for an improved physique or athletic performance. Bodybuilders are interested in muscle development as a means of enhancing their aesthetic appearance for competition. Weight lifters, power lifters, and other strength athletes are more interested in the ability to develop more strength and power. However, anabolic steroids may also stimulate the production of red blood cells (RBC), so they may be of interest to aerobic endurance athletes as a means of improving oxygen delivery to the muscles. Furthermore, steroids have been suggested to facilitate physiological recovery during intensive physical training on a daily basis, making them appealing to a variety of athletes.

One of the androgenic effects of anabolic steroids in some individuals is increased arousal and aggressiveness. These psychological changes have been suggested to help athletes train more intensely and thus develop their athletic physiological abilities to a greater extent.

Thus, a wide variety of athletes may use anabolic steroids for different theoretical reasons. The following section will discuss some of the research on their use and effectiveness as a means of enhancing various athletic performances.

Research Findings

Since the use of anabolic steroids by athletes has been and is so extensive, it has received considerable research attention. For our purposes we shall summarize the research findings in three areas, namely the extent of the use of anabolic steroids in sport, their effectiveness as a means of enhancing athletic performance, and the possible health risks associated with their use.

Use in Sport.   Weight lifters, power lifters, and bodybuilders appear to be the most prolific users of anabolic steroids. Reports from sports administrators and epidemiological surveys suggest that over 90 percent of the male athletes in these sports have used or will use steroids. The percentage is slightly lower among male field athletes (shot put, javelin, and discus) and football players, approximately 70 to 80 percent. Use is lower still in sprinters and decathletes, about 40 to 50 percent, and in endurance athletes, about 10 percent. The use of anabolic steroids by female athletes is considerably lower, ranging from 20 percent in strength athletes to only 1 percent in endurance athletes. In those athletic competitions in which drug testing has been initiated, the use of steroids appears to have diminished appreciably, at least as documented by the test results.

Although the therapeutic dose varies for the different anabolic steroids, a normal level is about 5 to 10 milligrams per day for the oral compounds. However, athletes have been reported to be taking anywhere between 10 and 300 milligrams daily, with reports as high as 2000 milligrams. Athletes also practice a technique called *stacking*, which involves the use of two or more different steroids at the same time, usually including testosterone as well as the oral and injectible steroids. Stacking may also involve a progressive increase in the types and dosages of steroids in order to obtain an optimal anabolic effect.

Survey research has shown that athletes often take other drugs in conjunction with anabolic steroids. Some drugs are taken to prevent some of the adverse side effects of steroids. For example, *human chorionic gonadotropin* (HCG) is used to prevent atrophy of the testicles, while *antiestrogens* are used to prevent development of the breasts in males. Other drugs such as *diuretics* may be used to reduce excessive water retention, and then potassium supplements are used to replace the potassium excreted by using diuretics. Female athletes may take *norethisterone*, normally found in birth-control pills, as a means of avoiding detection in drug testing. One author has characterized the use of two or more drugs at one time as the *polydrug abuse syndrome* among athletes.

Reports show that individual athletes adjust the use of steroids in preparation for competition in which they might be tested for drug use. Oil-based injectable steroids may be detected for months after use, whereas the oral steroids may be detectable for weeks. Thus, athletes will stop taking steroids some time prior to competition in order to avoid detection. Diuretics may also be used to expedite drug removal from the body. However, the sophisticated testing techniques developed for the Olympic games appear to have deterred steroid use at this level.

Because of this highly effective testing program, some athletes have turned to the anabolic agent of the future, *human growth hormone* (hGH). This agent is secreted by the pituitary gland to help support growth and development of body tissues. Not too long ago the only source of hGH was an extract from the pituitary gland. However, through genetic engineering a synthetic hGH was marketed in 1985. It has several bona fide medical applications, such as stimulating growth in a youngster with deficient natural sources of hGH, but it appears drug companies are attempting to produce more than is medically needed. Unfortunately, little research data are presently available relative to the effectiveness of hGH as a means of improving sports performance and its use in sport has not been thoroughly documented. However, this may change in the future if hGH becomes more readily available.

Effectiveness in Improving Sports Performance.   Researchers studying the effects of anabolic steroids on athletic performance have used several approaches. Much of the early research usually involved well-controlled experimental studies in laboratory surroundings so that the dosages, diets, and training programs could be controlled somewhat. However, as the health risks of steroid usage became more evident, researchers became reluctant to impose such risks upon human subjects, particularly if research was to be conducted with large doses. Thus, much of the recent research involves subjects, many of whom are athletes, who are already using steroids in training. Some of these subjects have been willing to alter their intake of steroids for the purposes of research. Although the data from these studies are not as valid as those from more controlled laboratory settings, often the results are still meaningful because they reflect actual steroid practices of the athletes.

The principal areas of interest to researchers have been body-composition changes, strength gains, and improvement in aerobic endurance. The first two involve the effect of anabolic steroids as a means of increasing muscle mass, whereas the latter involves the effect on RBC production. Although not all studies are in agreement about the effectiveness of anabolic steroids in improving performance associated with sport, the following summary is a rational interpretation of the available research and reflects conclusions published by the American College of Sports Medicine and the National Strength and Conditioning Coaches Association.

The general results of well-controlled studies and individual case studies strongly support the value of anabolic steroids as a means of increasing body weight, and the weight increase is due primarily to increases in lean body mass (muscle tissue) and not body fat. However, in order for steroids to be effective the athlete must be involved in a weight-training program and must increase protein intake to about two grams per kilogram of body weight per day. In a recent case study, one weight lifter following such a protocol increased his body weight by nearly 5 percent in 6 weeks when using steroids. The increases were attributed to gains in lean body mass and supported by measurement of body composition and biopsies of the muscles, which showed a significant increase in muscle fiber size. This athlete then continued to train for 6 weeks without steroids and experienced a drastic reduction in body weight and muscle fiber size, returning almost back to his original levels. It appears clear that anabolic steroids can help to increase muscle mass—but will they increase strength?

Over 50 percent of the well-controlled laboratory studies evaluating the effectiveness of anabolic steroids in improving strength and power have produced positive results. When averaging the results of several studies lasting between 10 and 15 weeks, subjects who took steroids improved their lifts by over 15 pounds in the bench press and over 20 pounds in the squat. The placebo group showed no such improvement. Most of the individual case studies have reported similar findings. In the case study cited above, the weight lifter experienced significant gains in strength over the 6-week period on steroids, but the strength gains vanished following the 6 weeks without steroids.

Although anabolic steroids may help to increase RBC production in individuals with certain types of anemia, they have not been shown to be effective in individuals with normal RBC levels. Moreover, eight studies have shown that anabolic steroids do not increase maximal oxygen uptake or aerobic endurance performance. Also, no evidence is available to support the contention that steroids will facilitate recovery in athletes, such as distance runners, who train at intense levels on a daily basis.

Health Risks.   Some of the health risks associated with anabolic steroids have been determined by studying patients who have used them for years. Often these findings are ignored by athletes because they do not believe the findings apply to them. However, recent data obtained from individuals who are self-administering anabolic steroids indicate some potential health problems. A number of these health problems are minor and do not pose any major health threat to the individual. Others, however, can be quite serious.

Anabolic steroids may effect several changes in physical appearance and personality that, although not serious health risks, may be discomfiting to some individuals. Acne, alopecia (baldness), growth of body hair, edema (accumulation of body water), breast enlargement in adult males and children of both sexes, as well as breast shrinkage, enlargement of the clitoris, and a deeper voice in adult females are some of the physical symptoms that have been reported. Mild personality changes, such as increased aggressiveness, have also been noted. However, some individuals have been reported to become extremely aggressive and hostile.

Because anabolic steroids are synthetic hormones, they may alter normal production and function of natural hormones in the body. Increased levels of anabolic steroids in the blood will depress the production of testosterone in males, leading to shrinkage of the testicles and a decrease in sperm production. Steroids also appear to increase the level of estradiol, a female sex hormone, in males, which may contribute to the development of female breast characteristics. Females taking steroids may experience irregularities in the menstrual cycle.

The use of anabolic steroids may pose some serious threats, particularly for women and children. Although many of the symptoms noted in the preceding two paragraphs are mild, temporary changes and have been shown to be reversible when steroid use is discontinued, several investigators have noted that some of the changes in females are irreversible. The use of steroids by children before the onset of puberty has been theorized to cause a premature fusion of the growth plate in the bones, leading to stunted growth.

The most serious health problems associated with steroid use are liver damage and the premature development of coronary heart disease. Several of the side effects of anabolic steroids will increase the risk for the premature development of *atherosclerosis*, the main cause of coronary heart disease and heart attacks. First, steroids can cause a retention of body fluids and

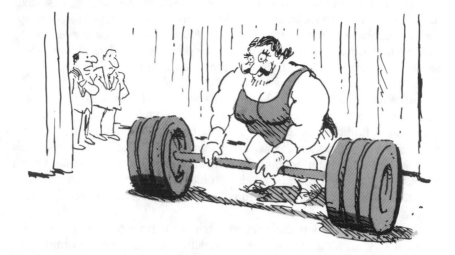

"I think we have to reduce her dosage."

sodium, which can lead to an elevated blood pressure. High blood pressure is a primary risk factor for atherosclerosis. Second, one of the characteristic findings of steroid use is a change in blood chemistry, namely a decrease in a form of cholesterol known as *high-density lipoprotein cholesterol* (HDL-C) and an increase in *low-density lipoprotein cholesterol* (LDL-C). This change in blood chemistry is unfavorable, as high levels of HDL-C and low levels of LDL-C are associated with a reduced risk for atherosclerosis. Third, steroids can contribute to clotting abnormalities in the blood that may precipitate the formation of a clot in the coronary arteries and blockage of blood flow to the heart muscle. Thus, the long-term use of steroids may predispose the athlete to an increased risk of cardiovascular disease.

Prolonged use of anabolic steroids has also been associated with severe liver damage. Research with animals has shown anabolic steroids to be weak *carcinogens*, that is, they are capable of causing cancer. Recent research with male bodybuilders suggests that steroids could suppress the immune system, which over a long period of time could increase the risk of cancer. About 40 cases are cited in the medical literature of humans who have developed either *liver cancer* or *peliosis hepatitis*, a condition characterized by blood-filled sacs in the liver that may rupture and cause serious complications or death. Although the vast majority of these individuals have been patients receiving steroids for treatment of medical problems, four recent case studies of liver cancer and cancer of the prostate gland have been associated with long-term steroid use in weight lifters and bodybuilders.

Finally, some of the other drugs used by athletes on steroids may also pose health risks. As noted previously, diuretics may cause excessive potassium losses, leading to decreased excitability in the heart muscle and possible fatal consequences. Human growth hormone may cause structural abnormalities in adults, particularly in facial bone development.

Recommendations

Legal, Ethical, and Medical Considerations. The use of anabolic steroids as a means of enhancing athletic performance cannot be recommended for several reasons. For one, steroids are banned by the IOC, NCAA, and most other sport-governing bodies and are therefore illegal in sport. Moreover, steroids appear to possess a high potential for medical abuse. Under no conditions should they be given to prepubescent athletes in attempts to improve performance. Possibly undesirable permanent changes in the physical appearance of females should discourage their use. The health risks noted for long-term users would appear to override any possible short-term benefits.

Nevertheless, despite the health-risk potential, athletes still use anabolic steroids in attempts to improve performance. To the thinking of many athletes, the potential short-term benefits do outweigh the potential long-term risks. Many athletes participate at a level of competition where there is no drug testing, so they do not have to worry about losing eligibility to play. For example, most high schools do not use drug testing. A large number of NCAA institutions do not have drug-testing programs in operation. In preparation for major competitions requiring drug testing, some athletes continue to take steroids, but, as mentioned previously, will use techniques in attempts to avoid detection. In an interesting recent development, the NCAA has decided to test for steroid use during training, not only for championship competition.

Because of the continued use of steroids by athletes, some physicians, several of whom are internationally recognized in sports medicine, have proposed that steroids be legalized for all athletes. They contend this would eliminate the unfair advantage one athlete may have over another. Also, they believe that with physicians controlling the prescription and monitoring the effect on the athlete through periodic blood tests, the various associated health risks may be avoided. However, one nationally prominent physician who formerly practiced this controlled use of steroids stopped when he discovered that the athletes he was serving were using large amounts of steroids obtained on the black market in addition to the ones he was prescribing. As noted previously, many athletes believe that if

1 pill is good, then 10 must be better. In fact, many athletes take 50 to 100 times the recommended dosage. Although the approach suggested by these physicians seems logical, it may not work in the real world of athletics. It is interesting to note that, as revealed by the chief medical officer for the United States Olympic Committee, nearly 30 to 40 percent of performance-enhancing drugs obtained by athletes come from physicians.

Other sports medicine physicians are recommending that anabolic steroids be listed as controlled substances, such as amphetamines, cocaine, and many of the depressants that come under federal control. Thus, prescriptions by a physician for nonmedical purposes, such as to a healthy athlete, or unregulated distribution would be grounds for criminal prosecution. Several states have already implemented such laws.

Athletes who do take anabolic steroids should be aware of the potential health risks. If they believe the benefits are worth the risks, they should at least have periodic blood tests by a knowledgeable physician to check for deteriorative changes in liver function and serum-cholesterol composition, as well as other health-risk factors.

Selected Readings

Books

Clarke, K. (Ed.). (1972). *Drugs and the coach.* Washington, DC: American Alliance for Health, Physical Education, and Recreation.

Goldman, B. (1984). *Death in the locker room.* South Bend, IN: Icarus Press.

Taylor, W. (1982). *Anabolic steroids and the athlete.* Jefferson, NC: McFarland.

Williams, M. (1974). *Drugs and athletic performance.* Springfield, IL: Charles C. Thomas.

Woodland, L. (1980). *Dope: The use of drugs in sport.* Newton Abbot, England: David and Charles.

Reviews

Beckett, A. (1981). Use and abuse of drugs in sport. *Journal of Biosocial Science,* **7**(Supplement), 163-178.

Bell, J., & Doege, T. (1987). Athletes' use and abuse of drugs. *The Physician and Sportsmedicine,* **15**(3), 99-108.

Biron, S., & Wells, J. (1983). Marijuana and its effect on the athlete. *Athletic Training,* **18**, 295-303.

Covert, J. (1986). Illicit drugs and the athlete. *American Pharmacy,* **26**, 39-45.

Cowart, V. (1988). Human growth hormone: The latest ergogenic aid. *The Physician and Sportsmedicine,* **16**(3), 175-181.

Duda, M. (1988). Study: Steroids lower immunity, lipids. *The Physician and Sportsmedicine,* **16**(2), 56-60.

Edwards, S., Glover, E., & Schroeder, K. (1987). The effects of smokeless tobacco on heart rate and neuromuscular reactivity in athletes and nonathletes. *The Physician and Sportsmedicine,* **15**(7), 141-147.

Eichner, E. (1986). The caffeine controversy: Effects on endurance and cholesterol. *The Physician and Sportsmedicine,* **14**(12), 124-132.

Era, P., Alen, M., and Rahkila, P. (1988). Psychomotor and motor speed in power athletes self-administering testosterone and anabolic steroids. *Research Quarterly for Exercise and Sport,* **59**, 50-56.

Fitch, K. (1986). The use of anti-asthmatic drugs. Do they affect sports performance? *Sports Medicine,* **3**, 136-150.

Glover, E., Edmundson, E., Edwards, S., & Schroeder, K. (1986). Implications of smokeless tobacco use among athletes. *The Physician and Sportsmedicine,* **14**(12), 95-105.

Haupt, H., & Rovere, G. (1984). Anabolic steroids: A review of the literature. *American Journal of Sports Medicine,* **12**, 469-484.

Ivy, J. (1983). Amphetamines. In M. Williams (Ed.), *Ergogenic aids in sport* (pp. 101-127). Champaign, IL: Human Kinetics.

Kepera, H. (1985). The history of anabolic steroids and a review of clinical experience with anabolic steroids. *Acta Endocrinologica Supplementum,* **271**, 11-18.

Kruse, P., Ladefoged, J., Nielsen, U., Paulev, P., & Sorenson, J. (1986). ß blockade used in precision sports: Effect on pistol shooting performance. *Journal of Applied Physiology,* **61**, 417-420.

Lamb, D. (1984). Anabolic steroids in athletics: How well do they work and how dangerous are they? *American Journal of Sports Medicine,* **12**, 31-38.

Lombardo, J. (1986). Stimulants and athletic performance (Part 1 of 2): Amphetamines and caffeine. *The Physician and Sportsmedicine,* **14**(11), 128-141.

Lombardo, J. (1986). Stimulants and athletic performance (Part 2 of 2): Cocaine and nicotine. *The Physician and Sportsmedicine,* **14**(12), 85-91.

Osneid, S. (1984). Doping and athletes: Prevention and counseling. *Journal of Allergy and Clinical Immunology,* **73**, 735-739.

Tesch, P. (1985). Exercise performance and ß-blockade. *Sports Medicine*, **2**, 389-412.

Van Handel, P. (1983). Caffeine. In M. Williams (Ed.), *Ergogenic aids in sport* (pp. 128-163). Champaign, IL: Human Kinetics.

Viitasalo, J., Kyrolainen, H., Bosco, C., & Alen, M. (1987). Effects of rapid weight reduction on force production and vertical jumping height. *International Journal of Sports Medicine*, **8**, 281-285.

Chapter 5

Physiological
Ergogenic Aids

IN THE PRECEDING CHAPTER we mentioned the case of an American swimmer in the 1972 Munich Olympic Games, who was deprived of his gold medal when drug testing revealed the presence of ephedrine, a stimulant found in medication he was taking for asthma. However, in the 1984 Olympic Games in Los Angeles several American cyclists were permitted to keep their gold medals even after admitting later to receiving blood transfusions prior to competition. Is there an inconsistency here?

Let us look again at the essential part of the International Olympic Committee (IOC) rule on doping.

> Doping is the administration of or the use by a competing athlete of any substance foreign to the body or of any physiological substance taken in abnormal quantity or taken by an abnormal route of entry into the body, with the sole intention of increasing in an artificial and unfair manner his performance in competition. When necessity demands medical treatment with any substance which because of its nature, dosage, or application is able to boost the athlete's performance in competition in an artificial and unfair manner, this is to be regarded as doping. (Clarke, 1972, p. 28)

By this definition it would appear that both situations just described would constitute doping. In the first case, *ephedrine* was specifically listed by the IOC as a banned drug, and even though it was being taken for medical purposes its use was illegal. In the second case, blood received via a transfusion seems to meet the criterion of a "physiological substance," but apparently in 1985, when this case evolved, blood transfusions were not specifically banned by the IOC, and there may have been some question as to whether abnormal quantities were taken, whether the blood was taken by an abnormal route of entry, or whether it was able to boost the athletes' performance in competition. These questions evidently have been resolved, however, as blood transfusions were banned by the IOC and the United States Olympic Committee (USOC) in 1985.

For the purpose of this chapter we shall consider physiological ergogenic aids as substances designed specifically to improve physiological processes that enhance human energy production. Physiological ergogenic aids are not drugs, so we might refer to them as physiological doping agents, or *nondrug doping*. However, they may be related to nutritional ergogenic aids, as several to be discussed in this chapter contain essential nutrients and could possibly have been discussed in chapter 3. On the other hand, several of the nutrients covered in chapter 3 might fit into the category of physiological doping agents. For example, vitamin C is a physiological substance and 10,000 milligrams is certainly an abnormal amount that some athletes may consume in an attempt to boost performance. As we shall see, several of the physiological aids to be discussed are banned for their possible ergogenic effect, whereas others are not banned and may be considered nutritional supplements.

Five different physiological aids will be covered in this chapter. *Oxygen supplementation*, *blood doping*, and *ingestion of carnitine* are theorized to improve energy production via the oxygen system; *ingestion of an alkaline salt*, such as *sodium bicarbonate*, is theorized to increase the capacity of the lactic acid energy system; and *phosphate salts* are theorized to benefit both energy systems.

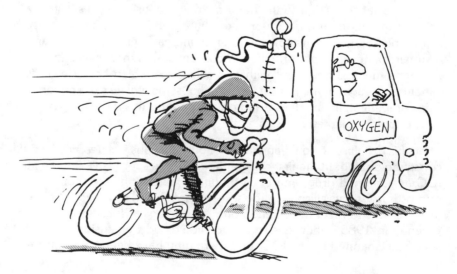

Oxygen Supplementation

Theoretical Basis

If you watch NFL football games on a regular basis, you will occasionally see a player on the sideline put a mask to his face and breathe deeply from a special gas tank. Such practices have also been observed in NCAA basketball championships. The air in the tank usually contains high amounts of oxygen; the players believe the oxygen may help to improve their performance. Is there any basis for this belief?

You may recall that in chapter 2 we noted that your body has three different energy systems to use during exercise and that the three systems are designed to produce ATP, the essential energy source for muscle contraction, at varying rates. The ATP-CP energy system is used primarily for short, powerful bursts of activity, whereas the lactic acid energy system also produces energy for slightly longer, yet still powerful, levels of exercise. Both of these energy systems are anaerobic—that is, they do not require oxygen in order to function. The third system, the oxygen system, is aerobic and does, of course, require oxygen. Although it cannot be itself used as a source of energy by the body during exercise, oxygen is necessary to help release the chemical energy stored in carbohydrates and fats in order to produce ATP for muscle contraction. In order to be successful, endurance athletes need to have highly developed oxygen energy systems.

Numerous studies have shown that aerobic endurance performance may be significantly impaired if the oxygen supply is limited, such as at high altitudes. A classic example of a field study with elite athletes was the 1968 Olympic Games, which were held in Mexico City at an altitude of 2,300 meters, or about 7,500 feet. Performances in events requiring anaerobic energy production were not adversely affected, but athletes in aerobic endurance events suffered considerable decrements in performance. Logical reasoning suggests that if low levels of oxygen, or *hypoxia*, decreases aerobic endurance, then oxygen supplementation, or *hyperoxia*, might enhance it.

Thus, the theoretical basis underlying the use of oxygen supplementation as an ergogenic aid is to increase the oxygen supply to the muscles in an attempt to improve energy production by the oxygen energy system. By improving ATP production via aerobic means, less ATP will need to be generated by the lactic acid energy system, decreasing the production of lactic acid that may contribute to the early onset of fatigue.

Research Findings

Research studies have used different procedures to administer oxygen, but the most common technique is to have subjects breathe air from a gas tank through a mouthpiece. The percentage of oxygen in the tank could be manipulated to range from the normal 21 percent, which would be the control or placebo condition, up to 100 percent. The effect of such oxygen supplementation techniques as a means of improving physical performance has been investigated in basically three different ways—before performance, after one performance in order to facilitate recovery for a subsequent performance, and during performance.

Oxygen Supplementation Prior to Exercise.   The ability to improve performance by breathing pure oxygen prior to a competitive athletic event does not appear to have much research support. In the first place, the blood has a limited capacity to store additional oxygen. The amount of blood in the average adult is about 5 liters, which contains about 1,000 milliliters of oxygen at rest. Breathing pure oxygen may increase this store by about 7 percent, or 70 milliliters, which is an insignificant amount relative to energy production. Also, unless the athlete were able to breathe the oxygen mixture immediately prior to competition, the small amount of extra oxygen would be dissipated in less than one minute of breathing normal air. Although some poorly designed studies nearly 80 years ago did show improvement in performance when oxygen supplementation was used beforehand, the results from better controlled contemporary research show no beneficial effects.

Oxygen Supplementation During Recovery.   One of the more popular uses of oxygen supplementation is to attempt to facilitate recovery during breaks in competitive athletic events. For example, athletes who are able to take periodic rest breaks due to the nature of their sport have all been known to use oxygen, such as track men between heats or football, basketball, and soccer players during substitutions and time-outs. Unfortunately for these athletes, several well-controlled studies do not support the value of this practice. The general design of these studies involved three phases. First, the athletes performed an exercise task comparable to those found in sports, such as maximal running speed for one minute, a series of fast sprints with short rest periods, or an endurance run to exhaustion on a treadmill. Next, the athletes rested for 10 to 30 minutes or so and breathed a gas mixture from a tank of either pure oxygen or a placebo of room air. Finally, the athletes repeated the exercise task. The investigators were usually interested in whether the oxygen was able to facilitate recovery by removing lactic acid at a faster rate or by improving performance on the second exercise task. In none of these studies was lactic acid removal or performance improved by the oxygen supplementation.

Oxygen Supplementation During Exercise.   On the other hand, oxygen supplementation during endurance exercise has been shown to improve physiological energy production and performance. Increases in maximal oxygen uptake have been reported to be about 2 to 5 percent due to the increased oxygen content in the blood. When breathing oxygen compared to room air was studied during a standard exercise task, such as running a mile at a 6-minute pace, the oxygen supplementation resulted in a lower heart rate, lower cardiac output, decreased breathing, and lower production of lactic acid. Thus, oxygen supplementation permitted runners to produce energy more efficiently, enabling them to run at a faster pace with the same physiological effort. A number of studies have shown that endurance performance is improved in a linear fashion with oxygen supplementation: The higher the percentage of oxygen in the supplement, the better the performance.

In summary, oxygen supplementation appears to be an effective ergo genic aid if administered during actual endurance performance, but will not improve performance when taken before competition nor facilitate recovery when taken after exercise.

Recommendations

Breathing Techniques.   Some investigators have suggested a possible application of oxygen supplementation prior to competition in short-distance swimming events, such as 50 meters. They have suggested that the oxygen might enable the swimmers to hold their breath longer and they might thus be able to swim the entire race without taking a breath. The idea is to prevent turning of the head to breathe, which may increase the body-surface area and resistance to forward motion. Unfortunately, this does not appear to be practical in actual competition unless the swimmer has a gas tank on the starting block. However, taking 5 to 10 deep breaths just before the start is practical and can increase breath-holding time substantially because those breaths help to lower blood levels of carbon dioxide, the main stimulus forcing you to breathe. Thus, this breathing technique may be more practical and effective than oxygen supplementation in this situation.

Some preliminary research has suggested another breathing technique, called breathplay, might help improve the efficiency of oxygen utilization during exercise. The study was conducted with bicyclists and involved specific breathing patterns, mainly a powerful exhalation followed by less forceful inhalations. The cyclists in the study who learned the breathplay technique improved several physiological functions, such as a delay in the onset of the anaerobic threshold and a lower heart rate during a standard exercise task. They also benefited psychologically, perceiving the exercise task as less stressful. The endurance performance of the bicyclists in this study also improved with breathplay. However, the authors did note that although the results are promising, more research is needed before breath-play can be regarded as an effective ergogenic aid. It may be that breathplay is a kind of psychological ergogenic aid. Such aids will be discussed in the next chapter.

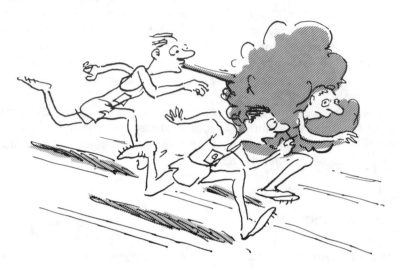

"I feel someone breathing down our necks."

You may wish to experiment with different breathing patterns involving forceful exhalations and more gradual inhalations; for example—runners may often use this technique—exhaling forcefully as one foot lands followed by inhalations on the next three foot plants. Other endurance athletes may pattern their breathing after the mechanics of their sport. A book by Ian Jackson, the developer of this technique, is in the reference list at the end of the chapter.

Legal, Ethical, and Medical Considerations.   As the available research strongly suggests that oxygen supplementation will not improve performance if taken before or during recovery periods in athletic competition, there appears to be little scientific logic to recommend its use as an ergogenic aid in these situations. Nevertheless, although oxygen supplementation under these conditions does not appear to be of any physiological value, some athletes may use it for psychological reasons. For example, NFL players may be aware that the atmospheric oxygen levels in Denver are lower than normal and thus may believe oxygen to be ergogenic. In such cases there may be no harm in providing oxygen supplementation, as its use is legal and, in the concentrations and amounts normally used in the NFL, it does not pose any medical risks. However, although we cannot dismiss the potential for improved performance through the psychological placebo effect, we should also be aware of the potential for decreased performance if the placebo is not available. For example, it is the last minute of the game, the score is tied, and the key running back, who believes oxygen is ergogenic, takes a big breath from the oxygen tank and finds it empty. The running back might be affected psychologically, and performance might suffer.

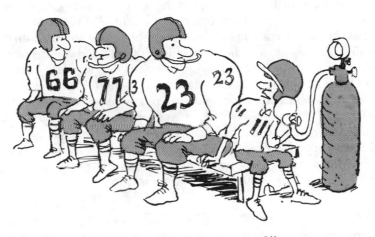

"Who used all the oxygen?"

Although oxygen supplementation during competition could be provided in a practical matter, such as strapping a lightweight tank to the chest of a bicyclist or transporting tanks on a bicycle or car next to a distance runner, such practices are illegal and, of course, cannot be recommended. Moreover, prolonged use of pure oxygen may lead to a condition of *oxygen toxicity* and actually depress ventilation.

Blood Doping

Theoretical Basis

It is interesting that much of the original research with ergogenic aids was conducted for military purposes. For example, the Germans conducted a number of studies with amphetamines, caffeine, and other stimulants during the 1930s regarding their effects on physical performance of a military nature, such as prolonged marching. During World War II the famous experiments conducted at the University of Minnesota explored the possibilities of nutritional supplements as ergogenic aids for military personnel. But one of the more interesting stories is the military rationale behind some of the earliest research with blood doping.

Military Applications.   In the latter stages of World War II American planes were increasing the number of bombing missions over Germany but suffering considerable losses from antiaircraft guns. One way of avoiding antiaircraft firing was to fly at higher altitudes, but the lower levels of oxygen at high altitudes disturbed normal functioning of the central nervous system, and the pilots and other crew members were more likely to make errors. In 1944-45, U.S. Navy researchers infused 1,300 milliliters of blood into two subjects and tested their physiological reactions at a simulated altitude of 18,000 feet. The subjects reacted favorably to the transfusion and were better able to tolerate the adverse effects of low oxygen levels at this altitude. The final report of this research was submitted in March, 1945; blood transfusions probably would have been used on U.S. aviators had the war not ended shortly thereafter. One of the findings of this early military research that revealed some possible application to sport was a lower heart rate response during exercise following the transfusion.

Blood Doping in Sports.   The theoretical basis for using blood transfusions to improve tolerance to low oxygen levels at high altitudes is the same for improving performance in sports, that is, to increase the oxygen-carrying capacity of the blood. The most common term used to describe this procedure in conjunction with athletics is *blood doping*, although other terms such as *blood boosting* and *blood packing* have also been used. Since RBC are also known as erythrocytes, the technical medical term for the procedure is *induced erythrocythemia*, or an induced increase in the number of RBC.

Blood doping can be achieved in several ways. One technique is *homologous transfusion*, or receiving the blood from another individual whose blood is compatible with yours. In this situation your normal RBC level is increased by the amount that is transfused. In the second method, known as *autologous transfusion*, you receive your own blood. In this method your blood has been withdrawn previously and stored for about 2 months while your body manufactures new RBC to return your RBC level to normal. In order to store your blood this long, the RBC are separated from the blood and frozen. Later they are thawed and mixed with a saline solution that facilitates transfusion. When whole blood or RBC in a saline solution is infused into your bloodstream your blood volume increases and causes an increase in blood pressure. This increase in blood pressure is not desirable, so your kidneys excrete excess plasma water, but the transfused RBC remain in the bloodstream. Thus, you experience an increased concentration of RBC.

As mentioned in a previous chapter, hemoglobin in the RBC is the primary means of transporting oxygen through the body. Thus, the theoretical value of blood doping in sport is simple. By increasing the RBC concentration and concomitantly the hemoglobin concentration, the blood is capable of transporting more oxygen to the muscle cells during exercise. Such a procedure should benefit athletes involved in competition where aerobic endurance capacity is important.

Although one of the principal investigators conducting research with blood doping in Sweden noted that its use among European athletes was rather widespread in the early 1970s, it was not until the 1976 Montreal Olympic Games that blood doping became an issue. Television commentators covering the Games suggested that the performance of several distance runners could have been enhanced by blood doping. Although the IOC was aware of the possible benefits derived from blood doping, nothing was done to prohibit its use in the 1980 Olympic Games in Moscow or the 1984 Games in Los Angeles. However, following the disclosure that several American cyclists used blood doping with apparent success in the 1984 Olympics, its use was banned in 1985. Nevertheless, because there is currently no test available to detect its use, evidence suggests that some endurance athletes continue to use blood doping for such major competitions as the New York City Marathon.

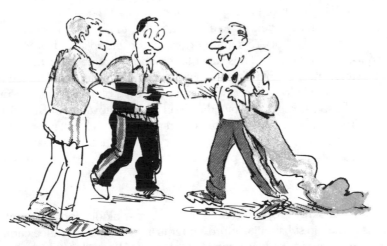

"Meet my new trainer. He specializes in hematology."

Research Findings

Much of the early research conducted with blood-doping techniques in the 1960s and early 1970s focused on physiological mechanisms of oxygen transport and factors that could limit maximal oxygen uptake. However, when the potential application of blood doping to sport became more evident, the research began to focus on its value as a means of improving athletic performance. In many of these later studies both the physiological effects and potential ergogenic effects of blood doping were investigated together.

Problems With Early Research.   The results of many of the studies conducted throughout the 1970s were contradictory. About half of the studies reported improved physiological functioning during exercise, such as an increased maximal oxygen uptake, whereas the remaining half revealed no improvements. Similar contradictory findings were noted relative to aerobic endurance capacity on exercise tests to exhaustion. However, careful analysis of the research revealed a major defect in the studies that were not finding any improvement in physiological functioning or endurance capacity. The general procedure in these studies involved the withdrawal of blood, storage in refrigeration for 21 days, and then reinfusion. The American Red Cross blood-donation regulations specify that refrigerated blood must be used within 21 days. However, 21 days is not ample time for the body to regenerate the RBC that have been lost through withdrawal. Thus, the subjects in these studies did not experience the significant increases in RBC levels or hemoglobin concentration necessary for improvement in maximal oxygen uptake and aerobic endurance.

Red blood cells that are separated from the blood and frozen can be stored for up to 3 years. Thus, as it takes about 8 weeks for the body to replace naturally the RBC lost following withdrawal, the use of frozen RBC is much preferable for subjects who use their own blood withdrawn previously. In those studies that allowed for complete restoration of RBC following withdrawal, the transfusion of blood did result in significant improvements in physiological functions. In some studies the increase in maximal oxygen uptake was about 10 to 15 percent.

Effectiveness With Proper Techniques.   Proper blood-doping techniques may also result in substantial improvements in aerobic endurance capacity, as shown by about 10 well-controlled studies. We will use a study conducted in our Human Performance Laboratory at Old Dominion University to illustrate our point. A local American Red Cross Blood Donation Center conducted all of the blood withdrawals and transfusions; the transfusions were autologous, as all subjects received their own blood. In this 6-month study, 12 highly trained long-distance runners each had a pint of blood removed on two occasions separated by 8 weeks, a total of approximately one quart of whole blood. The RBC were separated and frozen. About 6 weeks after the second withdrawal the subjects were trained for 2 weeks to run a 5-mile race for time on a treadmill in our laboratory. The subjects could control the pace of the treadmill, and their split times were given to them every half-mile so they would know their pace. At each half-mile they also reported how they felt psychologically by saying a number that corresponded to their *rating of perceived exertion (RPE)*.

At the completion of this training period, when their RBC levels were back to normal, they ran a 5-mile treadmill race to serve as a baseline. Five days later the RBC were mixed with saline to the equivalent of one quart of whole blood and infused into six of the subjects; the other six received an equivalent amount of saline solution as a placebo. Within 2 days another 5-mile race was performed on the treadmill. We then waited about 7 weeks for the RBC levels of those who had received the blood to return to normal. The subjects then ran the third 5-mile test, which also served as a baseline measure. Five days later the transfusion procedure was reversed, with the six subjects who received blood the first time now receiving the placebo and the first placebo group receiving their own blood.

The data were then organized by the four different conditions prior to the 5-mile time trials. The four trials were baseline pre-saline, post-saline, baseline pre-blood, and post-blood. Figure 5.1 illustrates the changes in the hemoglobin levels. Note the minimal difference in the three trials in which no blood was infused and the significant improvement following the blood transfusion. This increased hemoglobin level allows the runners to carry more oxygen to their leg muscles during the run. Figure 5.2 illustrates the 5-mile run time. Note that the results parallel the changes in the hemoglobin concentration, with the only significant difference being the faster time following the blood transfusion. On the average, the runners completed the 5 miles about 45 seconds faster with blood doping, or about 9 seconds per mile faster. We found also that although the subjects were running faster with blood doping, their feelings of psychological stress as measured by the RPE were significantly lower. A similar study conducted in San Diego about a year later revealed almost identical results, as runners completed 3 miles about 23 seconds faster, or 8 seconds per mile, following blood doping. If these results could be extrapolated to a 26.2-mile marathon the improvement would amount to about 3 to 4 minutes.

The available laboratory research provides strong support for the effectiveness of blood doping as a means of improving the performance of endurance athletes. One previous criticism of the research on blood doping was that all of the studies were done in a laboratory setting and might not be applicable in a field setting, such as an actual race. However, a recent study reported in the *Journal of the American Medical Association* revealed highly significant improvements in performance in a 10-kilometer race following blood doping, evidence that it may work in actual competition.

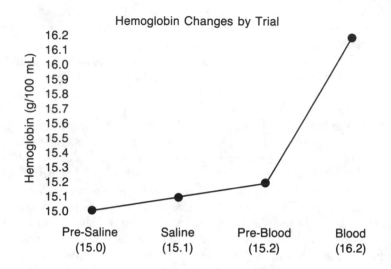

Figure 5.1   Hemoglobin increases following blood doping.

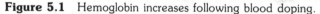

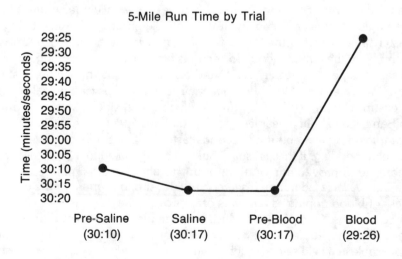

Figure 5.2   Runners improved their 5-mile times by an average of nearly 45 seconds following blood doping.

Recommendations

Legal and Ethical Considerations.   Although blood doping is one of the most effective ergogenic aids available, its use is illegal because it has been banned by the IOC and USOC. Furthermore, the American College of Sports Medicine has recently issued a position statement saying that the use of blood doping by athletes to improve performance is unethical.

However, anecdotal evidence in popular sport magazines suggests that some athletes may still be using blood doping in conjunction with events other than Olympic competition, such as major marathons and world championships. Fred Lebow, director of the New York City Marathon, was recently quoted as saying he was in favor of blood doping because a handful of athletes are using it, and that it is unfair to those who are not using it. One former American gold medal winner in the Olympic marathon recently noted in a popular runner's magazine that to do well in the Olympics, the minimum standard is to blood dope.

Although drug testing may be conducted following these events, there is currently no practical and accurate test available to detect the use of blood-doping procedures; researchers are attempting to develop such a test. Given the economic advantages of winning a major marathon and the social prestige associated with being a world champion, one may comprehend why athletes are using blood transfusions. Moreover, we may have a situation in upcoming Olympic Games comparable to the one that existed with anabolic steroids prior to the availability of effective drug-testing methods. Some athletes continued to use illegal anabolic steroids in Olympic competition when they knew their use would not be discovered.

Medical Considerations.   Improperly done, blood transfusions can be dangerous. For safety reasons, most transfusions in research studies are performed by physicians or other highly qualified medical personnel. From the popular sports journals it appears that elite athletes who are blood doping for competition are also under the care of physicians. One report noted that a physician for a national distance running team used blood transfusions for "therapeutic reasons," presumably to avert charges of unethical conduct in sports.

Under proper medical control the safest blood-doping procedure is the autologous transfusion, the infusion of the athlete's own blood that has been withdrawn previously and stored safely. There may still be problems with infections from the needle or injection of air into the blood stream, but these are rare with proper medical supervision. The amount of blood infused should be limited so that the *viscosity*, or thickness, of the blood does not become excessive. A high viscosity may lead to clotting within the blood vessels and possible heart failure. One quart of blood has been used successfully in several research studies, improving performance but not leading to excessive viscosity of the blood.

Homologous blood transfusions, the transfusion from a donor whose blood is compatible to the recipient, may be the source of medical risks in addition to the ones noted for autologous transfusions. One mild reaction to a homologous transfusion is the development of chills, fever, and nausea, which apparently struck several of the American cyclists prior to the 1984 Games, even though the blood they received was properly matched. More serious complications, even death, can occur if the blood is improperly matched. Another danger is that the donor's blood might contain several different virus types that may lead to such serious health problems as hepatitis, infection of the liver, or acquired immune deficiency syndrome (AIDS).

Thus, in addition to being judged illegal and considered unethical, blood doping as an ergogenic aid may be justifiably banned for medical reasons. Any athlete who desires to use blood doping should consider the possible consequences and should be under the supervision of qualified medical personnel.

Carnitine

Theoretical Basis

One of the newest theoretical ergogenic aids for sale is carnitine. Part of the reason for its recent popularity among some athletes may be the fact that in his book, Eat to Succeed, Robert Haas has recommended carnitine as an effective ergogenic aid. Although carnitine is an organic chemical compound produced in the body, most athletes have never heard of it.

Carnitine is found in most cells in the body, including the muscle cells, where its major function is to serve as a physiological carrier that facilitates the transport of fatty acids into the mitochondria (the energy powerhouses in the cells) for oxidation. Oxidation of fatty acids releases energy in the form of ATP. Theoretically, carnitine would be useful if it could increase the oxidation of fatty acids and spare the utilization of muscle glycogen (see Figure 3.4). You may recall that this is one of the theories underlying the use of caffeine as an ergogenic aid. Relative to this theoretical value, carnitine would be effective only for prolonged endurance events in which the sparing of muscle glycogen will provide for a more optimal fuel during the latter stages of the event.

Research Findings

Unfortunately, due to its recently realized potential as an ergogenic aid, carnitine has not received a great deal of research attention for this purpose. Research does reveal that carnitine levels rise in the blood during exercise. If carnitine was lost from the muscle the loss might impair fatty acid metabolism; however, investigators suggest that the liver is the source of the increased levels of carnitine in the blood, not the muscle tissues.

In one of the first controlled studies, Italian researchers fed 4 grams of carnitine per day for 2 weeks to trained long-distance walkers who then performed a series of laboratory tests on a treadmill. An unexpected finding in this study was a slight, but significant, increase in maximal oxygen uptake following the carnitine supplementation. On the other hand, the carnitine did not increase the use of fatty acids as an energy source during a 2-hour walk at 65 percent of $\dot{V}O_2max$. ($\dot{V}O_2max$, or maximal oxygen uptake, is one of the primary physiological measures of endurance capacity.) It also did not influence lactate production during an anaerobic exercise task. Both of these latter findings suggest that carnitine would not spare muscle glycogen stores.

Two recent reports released by researchers at Adelphi University in New York concluded that carnitine would not be an effective ergogenic aid. These well-controlled studies involved a double blind, placebo, crossover design with 10 physically conditioned subjects. The carnitine dosage was 500 milligrams daily for 28 days. One of the studies involved a maximal treadmill run to exhaustion and related physiological measures. In this study carnitine supplementation had no effect on running performance time or any of the physiological measures, including maximal oxygen uptake, maximal heart rate, anaerobic threshold, or maximal lactate levels. The other study involved a bicycle exercise task designed to achieve maximal aerobic work output for 60 minutes. Again, the use of carnitine did not increase the amount of work the subjects could do in one hour, nor have any influence on oxygen consumption, heart rate, or use of fatty acids as an energy source.

The limited research data available does not appear to support the value of carnitine as an effective ergogenic aid. However, one of the investigators has recommended that more research be conducted, particularly studies that might test the theoretical value of carnitine—that is, studies with prolonged endurance exercise where muscle glycogen sparing may be important.

Recommendations

Legal, Ethical, and Medical Considerations. Because there is very little support for the ergogenic value of carnitine there is also little basis to recommend its use. So far its use is legal, as it is not specifically banned by the IOC, but it would be possible to consider it a physiologial substance designed to improve performance (which might affect its legality as perceived by sport-governing authorities) if future research supports its effectiveness.

Investigators in the aforementioned research studies have not reported any medical risks or problems with the doses used. However, these investigators have used the *L-carnitine* preparation, not the *D-carnitine* or

DL-carnitine forms. Apparently the latter two forms of carnitine have a greater potential for toxicity, as supported by a medical case report of a long-distance runner who suffered an adverse reaction to their use.

Your decision whether or not to use carnitine as an ergogenic aid may be comparable to making a decision to use caffeine. If you are an endurance athlete involved in events that may benefit from the sparing of muscle glycogen, such as a full marathon, you may wish to test the theory of carnitine supplementation. It might be a good idea to start with the lower of the two doses used in research, 500 milligrams per day. Use only the L-form of carnitine. Unless you have access to blood tests and muscle biopsies, however, the only data you will have to test carnitine's effectiveness will be your time for a long-distance run, particularly the time for the last several miles. How you feel psychologically may also be recorded. But remember the placebo effect. You may do and feel better simply because you think you should. You can probably think of ways to control this, such as having a friend giving you either the carnitine or a placebo.

Finally, if you do decide to experiment with carnitine, do so during practice before trying it in competition.

Alkaline Salts

Theoretical Basis

If you ever took a basic chemistry class in high school or college you may recall working with strong acids, such as hydrochloric acid, which had the capacity to severely burn your skin. If such an accident occurred, the immediate first aid would be to wash the acid off, preferably with a neutralizing solution. You may be surprised to learn that certain cells in your stomach produce hydrochloric acid to aid in the digestion of dietary protein. Moreover, many of the physiological reactions in your body result in the formation of acids that could have serious consequences if not neutralized. For example, uncontrolled diabetes may lead to the formation of excessive amounts of acids from fat metabolism, which may lead to a series of events involving acidosis, diabetic coma, and death. In sports, lactic acid is related to the onset of fatigue in anaerobic events.

Acid-Base Balance.   Fortunately, your body produces certain substances known as *bases* that help to neutralize, or buffer, acids. These buffers that neutralize acids are often called *alkaline*. Much of the protein in your body may serve as an alkaline base; for example, hemoglobin in the RBC is a protein compound that is an excellent buffer of certain acids in the blood.

Your body must maintain a proper proportion of acids and bases; this proportion is usually referred to as *acid-base balance*. The acid-base balance in the body may be represented by the symbol *pH*, which basically represents the concentration of hydrogen ions in a solution. In essence, the more hydrogen ions in solution, the more acidic it is. Water, which is a neutral solution, has a pH of 7.0, whereas acidic solutions have a lower pH and basic solutions have a higher pH. Although this relationship seems contradictory, the mathematical method of determining pH is such that a low pH is associated with a higher concentration of hydrogen ions, or greater acidity.

The acid-base balance may vary in different parts of the body because certain enzymes function better in an acidic environment and others work better in a basic environment. Thus, gastric juices in your stomach are somewhat acidic (and may burn your esophagus when you belch and get heartburn) and those in your intestines are alkaline. Of importance to us is the pH of the blood and muscle cells.

The pH of the blood is about 7.3 to 7.4, or slightly alkaline, which appears to be an optimal level. Any deviation above or below this range for long periods of time can result in serious disturbances in normal physiological functioning, particularly in the brain. The diabetic coma resulting from *acidosis* (pH too low) is due to its effect on the brain. Thus, the body has a number of systems to control acid-base balance of the blood, including the proteins in your body cells and blood, your lungs (which blow off acid in the form of excess carbon dioxide), and your kidneys, which excrete acid salts. In addition, the blood contains a number of alkaline salts, most notably sodium bicarbonate, which can be used to rapidly buffer acids secreted into the blood.

Alkaline Salts and Sports Performance.   At rest the pH in the muscle cell is slightly alkaline, and the enzymes that produce energy via the lactic acid and oxygen energy systems appear to function optimally in this range. Exercise physiologists believe that if the concentration of hydrogen ions, and hence acidity, increases in the muscle cell then the optimal functioning of these enzymes will be disturbed and energy production will decrease. Thus, the onset of fatigue may occur due to the increased production of acid within the muscle cell when the lactic acid energy system is predominantly used during high-intensity exercise.

Basic research has revealed that the proteins within the muscle cell help to buffer metabolic acids during rest and exercise. However, beyond the initial buffering in the cell, the lactic acid produced during exercise appears to be buffered almost entirely by the sodium bicarbonate in the blood (see Figure 5.3). Thus, the theoretical basis underlying the ingestion of alkaline salts is to facilitate the removal of hydrogen ions from the muscle cell during exercise in order to help maintain the muscle cell near its optimal pH for enzyme functions and energy production.

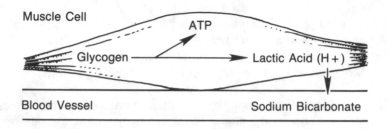

Figure 5.3 Alkaline salts are theorized to reduce the acidity in the muscle cell by facilitating the efflux of lactic acid.

The use of alkaline salts as an ergogenic aid is known by several different terms in the popular literature, including *buffer boosting*, *soda doping*, or *soda loading*. The soda term is derived from *baking soda*, which is *sodium bicarbonate*, the most commonly used alkaline salt for ergogenic purposes because of its easy availability. Other alkaline salts that have been used include *sodium citrate* and *potassium citrate*.

Alkaline salts are theorized to benefit athletes who rely heavily on the use of the lactic acid energy system during exercise. Classic examples are events in which athletes exert maximal anaerobic energy production for about 45 to 120 seconds, such as 400- to 800-meter runs in track or 100 to 200 meters in swimming, where lactic acid production is high. Since purely aerobic athletic events do not produce lactate rapidly in the muscle cell, alkaline salts have not been theorized to be of benefit to the endurance athlete.

Research Findings

Research with alkaline salts conducted over 50 years ago, both in Germany and the United States, revealed significant improvement in physiological measures associated with anaerobic exercise performance and in treadmill and bicycle ergometer exercise tests to exhaustion. Although this early research was supportive of an ergogenic effect and should have stimulated additional research, only a few studies were published in the next 40 years. In general, the results of these studies did not reveal any beneficial effects of alkaline salts upon performance in a 400-meter swim, a 1.5-mile run, or a treadmill run to exhaustion.

Research Designs.   In the last 10 years, however, there has been considerable research interest in alkaline salts as a means of reducing acidity in the muscle cell and improving anaerobic exercise performance. A variety of experimental designs have been used that involved differences in the exercise-testing procedures, the salts administered, and the physiological or performance measures recorded.

Most of the studies used exercise tasks that would stress anaerobic energy production via the lactic acid energy system, often with intermittent bouts of exercise and rest in order to see if the salts could facilitate recovery. These maximal exercise bouts were usually about 30 to 120 seconds long. Several studies used exercise tasks that were aerobic in nature in the early stages and gradually increased in intensity to become more anaerobic.

Different types of salts were given also. Some were alkaline. The placebo was usually a neutral salt that would not change the acid-base level, but in some studies acid salts actually were given to increase the acidity of the blood. Some studies used different alkaline salts and different dosages, but the most commonly used was 200 to 300 milligrams of sodium bicarbonate per kilogram of body weight. For an average male of 70 kilograms (154 pounds), this would amount to about 3 to 4 level teaspoons of baking soda.

Physiological Effects.   Investigators usually took a number of different measurements, such as blood pH, blood lactate (the form that lactic acid takes in blood), the amount of work produced in a set time such as 30 to 120 seconds, the power produced in 5 seconds, the exercise time to the point of fatigue or exhaustion, and the psychological stress of the exercise task as measured by ratings of perceived exertion (RPE). Several studies used muscle biopsies to look at changes in muscle pH.

Over 20 different well-controlled studies have been conducted recently with alkaline salts. The results are not in total agreement, as might be expected with such differences in experimental design.

One common finding is that alkaline salts will increase the pH of the blood before the exercise test and that this increased *alkalinity* (increased pH) will still be present following the test. Theoretically, this should facilitate the efflux of hydrogen ions and lactic acid from the muscle cell. However, research findings relative to blood lactate and muscle pH levels are mixed. If alkaline salts facilitate the removal of lactic acid from the muscle, then the amount of lactic acid should be higher in the blood. Although some studies support this effect, an equal number do not. Moreover, the data regarding the effect of alkaline salts on muscle pH are also equivocal, with one study reporting no change and another showing a significant increase compared to the control condition, an indication that the alkaline salts were effective in facilitating lactic acid release.

Psychological Effects.   Several studies used the RPE to evaluate psychological stress while subjects were working at a standardized exercise workload. The findings of these studies are in general agreement. When the exercise intensity of the workload was below 60 percent of maximal oxygen uptake, alkaline salts had no effect on the RPE. However, when the workload was increased to above 80 percent of maximal oxygen uptake, which would become partly anaerobic for most subjects, the RPE values were lower following the ingestion of alkaline salts, indicating that the subjects perceived the workload to be less strenuous.

Performance Effects.   These studies suggest alkaline salts may exert a beneficial psychological effect during exercise. The research findings relative to improved exercise performance are also supportive, although not totally. Improvements have been noted in laboratory studies with such tasks as the amount of work accomplished in 30 to 120 seconds, exercise tests to exhaustion on a bicycle ergometer or treadmill up to 10 minutes in duration, and performance on anaerobic tasks after prolonged aerobic exercise. In addition, one well-designed field study reported a significantly faster running time, about 2.9 seconds faster, for 800 meters in varsity track athletes.

Contrariwise, other laboratory studies using similar tests have revealed no significant improvement. Moreover, peak power output in short-term exercise tasks, such as 5 seconds, has not been improved with alkaline salts. In essence, however, the results are almost evenly divided, with about half of the studies finding significant ergogenic effects of alkaline salts and the other half reporting no improvement.

It may be important to note that no negative effects on performance have been reported—that is, in no study did physical performance decrease.

Recommendations

Whether or not alkaline salts improve performance is debatable, but because nearly half of the studies have revealed positive results, about half have found no improvement, and no studies have found a decrease in performance, logic suggests they may be helpful to some individuals if used properly.

It appears alkaline salts are best suited for athletes using the lactic acid energy system in sports demanding all-out effort for periods of about 30 seconds to 5 minutes, although the lactic acid energy system may also be involved in activities of lesser and greater time periods than this range.

Sodium bicarbonate, or baking soda, is readily available, but sodium and potassium citrate may also be used. An adequate dose would be about 300 milligrams, or 0.3 grams, per kilogram (2.2 pounds) of body weight.

Simply calculate your body weight in kilograms (by dividing your weight in pounds by 2.2) and then multiply by 0.3 grams. For a 176-pound athlete, the amount of sodium bicarbonate would be 24 grams ($176/2.2 = 80$; $80 \times 0.3 = 24$). This would be about five level teaspoons, as a level teaspoon holds about 5 grams. The bicarbonate can be mixed in enough water or other beverage to make it palatable and then should be consumed on an empty stomach approximately 30 to 60 minutes before exercise.

A possible alternative to alkaline salts is the consumption of large amounts of foods that are alkaline in nature. Fruit juices, in particular, are high in potassium citrate.

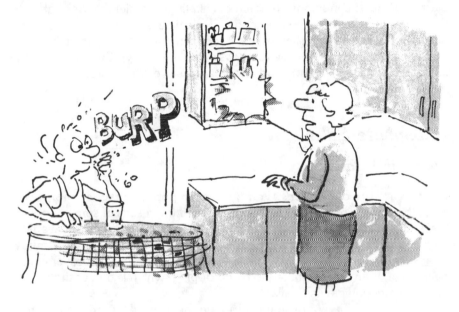

"I could swear I just bought a new box of baking soda."

Legal and Ethical Considerations.   Alkaline salts appear to be one of those ergogenic aids on the borderline in regard to legality. At the present time their use to improve performance does not appear to be specifically banned by the IOC, although they could be classified as physiological substances in a similar vein as blood doping. On the other hand, they may be regarded as a nutrient designed to increase the natural level of alkaline salts in the body. Looked at in this way, soda loading might be considered comparable to carbohydrate loading.

Although the use of alkaline salts may not be banned for ergogenic reasons, they should not be used by athletes who will be competing in events that test urine for drugs. Just as alkaline salts make the blood more alkaline, so too will the acidity of the urine be lowered, which will interfere with the validity of the tests for various drugs. In such a case the use of alkaline salts might be seen as an attempt by the athlete to avoid detection of the use of drugs and could lead to disqualification.

Medical Considerations.   As with any other legal ergogenic aid that you might try, it is best to try an alkaline salt in practice before using it in competition. Many of the subjects in the research studies experienced some form of gastrointestinal distress about 60 minutes after ingesting the bicarbonate solution. Many subjects developed diarrhea, and one investigator noted that several of his subjects had what he termed "explosive diarrhea." Such conditions could be debilitating in athletic performance. Furthermore, excessive consumption of alkaline salts may lead to the development of a severe alkalosis (pH is too high), which may disturb neurological functioning comparable to acidosis (pH is too low). Symptoms may include irritability, delirium, and possible spasm of the muscles.

Phosphate Salts

Theoretical Basis

In a recent issue of *Runner's World*, the most popular magazine for runners, the authors of one article theorized that if the results of some current research could be applied to runners, the use of phosphate salts would improve the performance of a 3-hour marathoner to 2:45 and a 40-minute 10-kilometer runner to 34:20. This would be a phenomenal improvement, even better than that attributed to blood doping, which is one of the most effective ergogenic aids available.

Like alkaline salts, phosphate salts have been used as ergogenic aids for well over 50 years. Some early German research suggested that phosphate salts could increase work productivity. There are reports they were used by German soldiers in World War I to relieve fatigue. Other German research in the 1930s suggested phosphate salts may improve sports performance. They consequently became commonly used by European athletes, a popularity that persists today. Their ergogenic qualities are still advertised in European sports journals. One commercial phosphate salt supplement available in the United States, *Stim-O-Stam*, is also marketed for athletes and advertised as an ergogenic aid to enhance endurance and reduce recovery time.

Results of both the dated and the contemporary research with phosphate salts suggest that they may be used by track athletes in events ranging in distance from the 100-meter dash to the 26.2-mile marathon. To be effective over this wide range, the phosphate salts would have to have the potential to improve energy production in all three human energy systems—the ATP-CP, lactic acid, and oxygen systems.

Phosphorus is an essential nutrient in the diet. In your body phosphorus is present as phosphate salts. The vast majority of phosphates are combined with calcium to form calcium phosphate, which serves as a structural basis for bones and teeth. Phosphates are also bound to other chemicals in the body that have important physiological functions relative to energy production.

Relative to the ATP-CP energy system, phosphates form high-energy bonds when attached to the organic compounds adenosine (ATP) and creatine (CP). Sodium and potassium phosphates serve as buffers in the body and may function similarly to alkaline salts in improving the lactic acid energy system. They may also benefit the oxygen energy system in several ways. Phosphates are necessary for optimal functioning of several B vitamins, such as B_1 (thiamine), which is involved in aerobic energy production from carbohydrates and fats. Also, phosphates are part of a compound found in the RBC known as *2,3-DPG (2,3-diphosphoglycerate)*, which facilitates the release of oxygen from hemoglobin to the muscle cells (see Figure 5.4).

Theoretically then, phosphate salts could be used to benefit performance over a wide range of athletic endeavors if they could increase the physiological potential of each of the three human energy systems. The use of phosphate salts for ergogenic purposes has also been called *phosphate loading*.

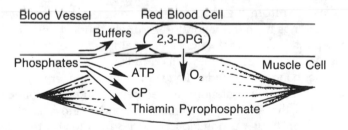

Figure 5.4 Phosphates have several possible roles in energy processes.

Research Findings

Early Research.   The early German research that served as a basis for recommending phosphate salts as an ergogenic aid to athletes has been reviewed extensively. As with most dated research with ergogenic aids the experimental designs of the studies were not well controlled, so many times the results were attributed to a placebo effect and were not considered valid. Nevertheless, in one of the earliest reviews of the research data a prominent Scandinavian researcher in 1939 concluded that if taken in quantities exceeding the amounts found in the normal diet, phosphate salts could probably increase human energy production.

Contrasting Findings in Contemporary Research.   For some reason there was little research conducted with phosphate salts and physical performance in the following 40 years. Then in the mid-1980s a research report generated at the University of Florida renewed interest. In this well-controlled study (a double-blind, placebo, crossover design), 10 highly trained distance runners consumed 4 grams of sodium phosphate for 3 days prior to exercise testing. The authors noted that the phosphate salts increased the level of 2,3-DPG in the blood and that this increase correlated with the increase noted in maximal oxygen uptake, about a 6 to 12 percent increase. The amount of lactic acid produced during a submaximal level of exercise was also reduced, which the authors attributed to an increased oxygen delivery to the muscle tissues. Moreover, although no running performance data was reported, the authors did note that the subjects ran longer on the treadmill after receiving the phosphate salts.

Other research findings from the Florida physiology laboratory appearing in the scientific and popular literature suggest that phosphate salts will reduce the perceived psychological stress, as measured by RPE, of riding a bicycle for 3 hours at 75 to 80 percent $\dot{V}O_2$max. Physiological measurements during this study suggested that increases in 2,3-DPG improved the release of oxygen from the RBC and thus reduced the workload of the heart. The findings from this laboratory strongly support an ergogenic effect of phosphate salts, and the lead investigator in these studies has been quoted as saying that phosphate salts do allow for better performance.

On the other hand, other studies have not revealed any ergogenic benefits of phosphate salt supplementation. Researchers at Brigham Young University investigated the effect of a commercial phosphate salt supplement (Stim-0-Stam) on power production, a 2 to 3 minute run to exhaustion on a treadmill, and recovery from these tests of power and anaerobic endurance. In essence, they were studying the effect of the phosphate salts upon the ATP-CP and the lactic acid energy systems. The results revealed no significant benefit of the Stim-O-Stam on any of the performance tests or on recovery. A research group at Adelphi University conducted several studies regarding the effect of phosphate loading on the oxygen energy system. In contrast to the University of Florida researchers, they found no beneficial effect of the salts on maximal oxygen uptake, lactate production, or performance on an 8-kilometer (5-mile) bike race.

Recommendations

Legal, Ethical, and Medical Considerations.   Comparable to the results of the research with alkaline salts, the effectiveness of phosphate salts to improve physical performance is debatable. Their use by athletes appears to be legal, for they are not specifically banned at the present time, although they could be considered a physiological substance when taken in a quantity that improves physical performance. Excesses of phosphorus in the body are normally excreted in the urine, so the use of phosphate salts as currently practiced does not appear to pose any significant medical risk. However, excesses in phosphorus combined with low levels of dietary calcium may contribute to a calcium deficiency.

Athletes desiring to experiment with phosphate salts may use the regimen practiced by the researchers at the University of Florida. It was successful for them and no adverse effects in the subjects were reported. The dosage was 1 gram of sodium phosphate taken four times per day, or 4 grams per day, for 3 to 4 days prior to competition. The last dose may be 2 to 3 hours prior to the event. As previously noted, try any ergogenic aid in practice before using it in competition.

Selected Readings

Books

Clarke, K. (Ed.). (1972). *Drugs and the coach.* Washington, DC: American Alliance for Health, Physical Education, and Recreation.

Haas, R. (1986). *Eat to succeed.* New York: Rawson Associates.

Jackson, I. (1986). *The breathplay approach to whole life fitness.* New York: Doubleday.

Morgan, W. (1972). *Ergogenic aids and muscular performance.* New York: Academic Press.

Williams, M. (Ed.). (1983). *Ergogenic aids in sport.* Champaign, IL: Human Kinetics.

Reviews

American College of Sports Medicine. (1987). Position stand on blood doping as an ergogenic aid. *Medicine and Science in Sports and Exercise,* **19**, 540-543.

Berglund, B., Hemmingsson, P., & Birgegard, G. (1987). Detection of autologous blood transfusions in cross-country skiers. *International Journal of Sports Medicine,* **8**, 66-70.

Boje, O. (1939). Doping. *Bulletin of the Health Organization of the League of Nations, 8*, 439-469.

Brien, A., & Simon, T. (1987). The effects of red blood cell infusion on 10-km race time. *Journal of the American Medical Association, 257*, 2761-2765.

Burfoot, A., Harmon, J., & Shafquat, S. (1986). One step beyond. *Runner's World, 21*(10), 49-52.

Burfoot, A., & Hirsch, G. (1987). Coming of age. *Runner's World, 22*(12), 56-61.

Carlin, J., Reddan, W., Sanjak, M., & Hodach, R. (1986). Carnitine metabolism during prolonged exercise and recovery in humans. *Journal of Applied Physiology, 61*, 1275-1278.

Duffy, D., & Conlee, R. (1986). Effects of phosphate loading on leg power and high intensity treadmill exercise. *Medicine and Science in Sports and Exercise, 18*, 674-677.

Eichner, E. (1987). Blood doping: Results and consequences from the laboratory and the field. *The Physician and Sportsmedicine, 15*(1), 121-129.

Gledhill, N. (1984). Bicarbonate ingestion and anaerobic performance. *Sports Medicine, 1*, 177-180.

Gledhill, N. (1985). The influence of altered blood volume and oxygen transport capacity on aerobic performance. *Exercise and Sport Sciences Reviews, 13*, 75-93.

Hommen, N., Cade, R., Privette, M., & Dippy, J. (1988, January). Effect of PO_4 and various field replacement regimen on blood volume (BV), cardiac output (Q_C), and endurance during bicycle exercise. (Abstract). Paper presented at the conference of the Southeast Chapter of the American College of Sports Medicine, Winston-Salem, NC.

Morris, A. (1983). Oxygen. In M. Williams (Ed.), *Ergogenic aids in sport* (pp. 185-201). Champaign, IL: Human Kinetics.

Nash, H. (1988). L-carnitine: Unproven as an ergogenic aid. *The Physician and Sportsmedicine, 16*(3), 74-75.

Welch, H. (1987). Effects of hypoxia and hyperoxia on human performance. *Exercise and Sport Sciences Reviews, 15*, 191-221.

Chapter 6

Psychological Ergogenic Aids

IN A RECENT INTERVIEW FOLLOWING a world-championship boxing match, the loser, a victim of a fifth-round technical knockout, had this to say: "I was very tight going into the fight. I felt tight the last few days. I couldn't relax. I'd try to relax, but I couldn't. I felt I couldn't get a deep breath. I felt like I was a step behind the whole night. Everybody handles pressure differently." Although this boxer's body was probably ready for the fight, his mind was definitely not ready. In sports, the mind and body depend on each other for optimal functioning. What affects the body can affect the mind, but also what affects the mind can affect the body.

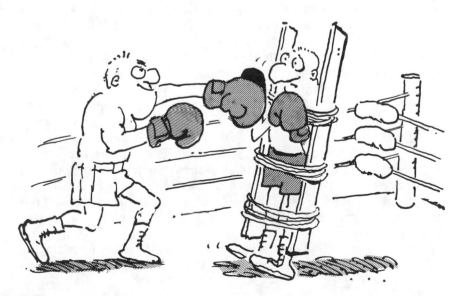

The thrust of this book has been on energy production during exercise; up to this point we have focused primarily on physiological energy production by the three human energy systems as a means of producing movement in sports. In sports, the human energy systems represent the *body*. As noted previously, you have inherited a given capacity for each energy system, but you need to maximize that system through proper physical training. Up to now we have stressed those ergogenic aids designed to enhance physiological energy production. For example, endurance athletes might use such nutritional aids as carbohydrate loading to provide an optimal fuel supply, such pharmacological aids as caffeine to help regulate the use of carbohydrate, and such physiological aids as blood doping to increase the oxygen supply for carbohydrate oxidation. Athletes will not be able to perform at an optimal level unless their physical energy systems are functioning at their best.

As noted in the introductory chapters, however, the human energy systems and support systems activated during exercise are ultimately controlled by the brain and spinal cord, collectively known as the *central nervous system*. Most of the neural control, or motor control, of your human energy systems to produce movement functions at a subconscious level. For example, when you begin to jog, hundreds of different muscles contract in rhythm, but you do not have to think about contracting each one at a specific time. Your nervous system will call each muscle into play at the appropriate time and also control the rate of energy production by the appropriate energy systems. In addition, the support systems for energy production are precisely regulated by the *autonomic nervous system*, a branch of the central nervous system. In this regard the rate and force of your heart contractions, as well as other body functions, adjust automatically to meet the demands of the exercise task. Thus, many times during such exercise as long-distance running you can put your body into automatic pilot and think about other things.

On the other hand, many times in sport you have to be very conscious of what you are doing, such as when you are at bat awaiting a pitch. In such a situation, the motor control portion of your brain needs to be functioning at an optimal level. It has to receive information, interpret it rapidly, and make a quick decision. There are three aspects to this process. First, how effectively do your senses receive the appropriate information or input? Second, how rapidly do the analytical parts of your brain interpret this visual information? And third, how accurately does the motor control portion of your brain activate the right muscles with the appropriate amount of force for optimal output? Any defect in the input or interpretation phase of this motor control process will lead to less than the optimal output (see Figure 6.1).

In one way or another your brain controls virtually every physiological activity in your body. Although you rarely exercise its full potential, you

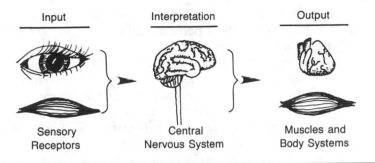

Input	Interpretation	Output

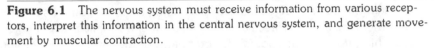

| Sensory Receptors | Central Nervous System | Muscles and Body Systems |

Figure 6.1   The nervous system must receive information from various receptors, interpret this information in the central nervous system, and generate movement by muscular contraction.

can train your brain to an extraordinary degree. For example, you can learn to control parts of your brain (including the autonomic nervous system) to the extent that you may lower your heart rate, decrease your blood pressure, increase blood flow to an area of your body, or change your skin temperature simply by thinking about such developments. You can also train the motor control center in your brain to exert very precise regulation of your muscular system. You can learn to make any individual muscle contract, such as wiggling your ears or moving your middle toe only. Furthermore, many of the maneuvers in sports, such as gymnastics, attest to the ability of the brain to control complex muscular movement patterns as well.

But the functioning of the motor control area may be influenced by a part of the brain that you have not trained or by neural feedback from parts of the body. Your conscious thoughts, your emotional feelings, and your perceptions of bodily sensations experienced during athletic competition may either enhance or impair your performance. It is in this sense that we discuss the importance of the psychological state of the mind in sport; for although the mind controls the body, the functions of the mind are also susceptible to control.

It is interesting that some of the ergogenic aids previously discussed may have some important implications for neural or psychological functioning during sport. As a nutritional aid, carbohydrate intake can prevent the adverse effects that low blood glucose levels have on brain function. Pharmacological aids such as stimulants and depressants may exert direct effects on brain function. Physiological aids may benefit metabolic processes in the muscle cells that normally lead to psychological stress; for example, the use of alkaline salts to buffer lactic acid and help decrease acidosis in the blood and subsequent mental discomfort. Thus, some ergogenic aids may improve sport performance by benefiting both physiological and psychological processes important to success.

As noted in chapter 1, you are confronted with a number of barriers in attempts to achieve your optimal performance in sports. In the next chapter we shall discuss mechanical constraints, but for now let us briefly review physiological and psychological barriers. Let us suppose that your biceps muscle has the physiological potential to lift 400 pounds. That is, if your ATP-CP energy system could be maximally activated, the force developed would be transmitted to your forearm bone to move the weight. Unfortunately, such a force could prove to be excessive and could actually pull away a piece of the bone, a condition known as an *avulsion fracture*. Although avulsion fractures do occur in such sports as weight lifting and arm wrestling, they are rare because of psychological limitations. Psychological barriers are inbuilt protective mechanisms that normally prevent you from reaching your full physiological potential. For example, in this case your psychological limits may permit you to lift only 100 pounds.

Just as you have inherited a set of physical and physiological characteristics that may predispose you to success in a given sport, so too have you inherited a variety of psychological characteristics of similar value. Moreover, physical training can improve both physiological and psychological characteristics important to sport. For example, proper training will allow the lactic acid energy system in your muscles to produce more energy, but your psychological tolerance to pain will also increase, allowing you to accumulate more lactic acid in the blood prior to the onset of fatigue. Your psychological limits have been raised. Although physical training in itself can help to raise your psychological limits, psychological ergogenic aids are theorized to augment them even more.

Before we turn our attention to specific psychological ergogenic aids, let us look at the relationship between arousal and psychological energy and at how mental training might help us to control our psychological energy in a manner comparable to the effect physical training has on our physiological energy production.

Arousal and Psychological Energy

The use of various psychological ergogenic aids to improve athletic performance may depend on the nature of the sport. Before we look at some specific methods, let us review several of the basic theories underlying the role of psychological energy in sport. For our purposes we shall think of *psychological energy as the level of arousal* experienced by the athlete, which may range on a continuum from deep sleep to an extreme state of excitation.

The Drive and Inverted U Theories of Arousal

The *drive theory* proposes that performance and arousal are directly related. That is, as your level of arousal is increased, so too is your performance. This theory may be supported in athletic events that contain relatively basic, simple movement patterns, such as weight lifting. As illustrated in Figure 6.2, the higher the degree of psychological energy, or arousal, the greater the strength potential.

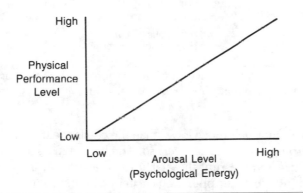

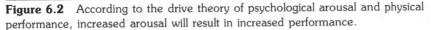

Figure 6.2   According to the drive theory of psychological arousal and physical performance, increased arousal will result in increased performance.

For sports that involve complex movement patterns and thought processes, the *inverted U theory* presented in Figure 6.3 may be more relevant. This theory proposes that there is an optimal level of arousal, which in Figure 6.3 is theorized to be a moderate level. Arousal levels that are either too low or too high may interfere with optimal performance. For example, a basketball team that reads in the paper that they are favored by 30 points may enter the game with a low level of arousal, believing all they have to do to win is show up for the game. They may not get aroused until they are down by 10 points in the last few minutes of the game, and by then it may be too late. On the other hand, if the same team is a 30-point underdog they may get so aroused that their high anxiety level actually impairs their ability to dribble and shoot the ball effectively.

The inverted U theory may be applied to a wide variety of sports, and athletes may find themselves on either end of the U continuum for various reasons. Athletes who have high levels of ability but face little challenge or demand are less likely to become aroused and more likely to be bored. They may suffer losses in concentration and drive and are thus more likely to suffer an upset in competition. On the other end of the continuum,

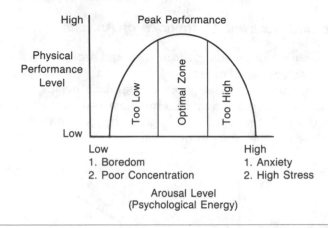

Figure 6.3 According to the inverted U theory of psychological arousal and physical performance, an optimal level of arousal will result in peak performance.

athletes with ability levels much lower than the challenge they face are more likely to be aroused, often excessively so. The high anxiety and stress levels they experience may disrupt the ability to concentrate, increase muscle tension, and induce other physiological changes that may impair performance. Whenever the arousal level of the athlete is too low or too high, psychological ergogenic aids can be used to move athletes towards more optimal arousal levels, or zones.

Optimal Arousal Zones

It is important to note that the *optimal arousal zones* may vary for different sports. For example, Figure 6.4 represents theoretical curves for three sports—archery, tennis, and weight lifting. In archery the optimal arousal

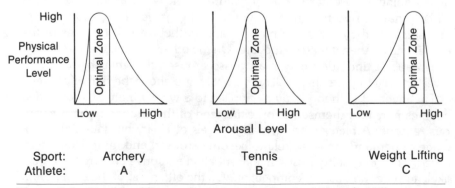

Figure 6.4 Possibly, differences exist in optimal arousal zones for different sports or different athletes.

zone might be low because any increase in muscle tension could result in an impaired accuracy. In tennis either too little or too much arousal could adversely affect performance, so the optimal zone is in the middle. In weight training the higher the arousal level the better, but there could be a point where excessive anxiety might disrupt concentration.

The optimal arousal zone may also vary for different athletes. The curves in Figure 6.4 could represent three different batters. Each batter performs best with a different arousal level. The optimal arousal level for batter A is low, for batter B it is medium, whereas batter C needs a high level.

The key to using psychological ergogenic aids is to know where your optimal arousal zone is located. For any athlete this zone may change depending on the competition and the importance of the contest. Thus, you need to know yourself and how you react to different levels of athletic competition. If you do know yourself, then the use of various behavior-modification techniques (also known as psychological ergogenic aids) may help to improve your performance.

Mental Training and Psychological Ergogenic Aids

As we have noted previously, one of the most effective ways to improve athletic performance is through proper physical training. Depending on the sport, there are a wide variety of training options available. For example, for distance runners such techniques as interval training, repetition running, long-distance running, anaerobic threshold training, fartlek, and others have been used successfully.

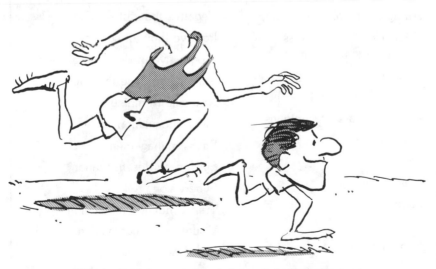

Physical and mental training are both important.

Several years ago I initiated a running program for myself, mainly to maintain body weight and cardiovascular fitness. Eventually, though, I began to participate in local road races. One year I decided to concentrate on improving my times. As I perused several running magazines throughout the year I found over a half-dozen training programs specifically tailored for 10-kilometer (6.2 miles) races that were used by some of the top runners in the world. An analysis of the training programs revealed many differences, but there was a thread of commonality among them. Basically the programs were designed to increase maximal oxygen uptake and to raise the anaerobic threshold, or, in essence, to maximize the positive value of aerobic energy production and minimize the negative aspects of lactic acid accumulation.

The psychological ergogenic aids discussed in this chapter are in reality forms of mental training and are somewhat analogous to physical training. A review of the sport-psychology literature reveals a wide variety of mental-training approaches or techniques that may be used with athletes, many of which are listed in Table 6.1. In general, just as physical training

TABLE 6.1
**SOME PSYCHOLOGICAL ERGOGENIC AIDS
APPLIED TO SPORT**

Attention control training	Mental dissociation
Attributional retraining	Mental rehearsal
Autogenic training	Negative thought stopping
Cognitive affective stress management training	Positive thought control
	Progressive muscular relaxation
Cognitive restructuring	Rational emotive therapy
Concentration training	Relaxation training
Covert rehearsal techniques	Stress inoculation
Flooding	Stress management
Flow	Systematic desensitization
Goal setting	Sybervision
Hypnosis	Transcendental meditation
Imagery	Visual motor behavior rehearsal
Implosive training	Water flotation tanks

is designed to maximize the positive aspects and minimize the negative aspects of physiological energy production, so too does mental training attempt to maximize positive psychological energy and minimize negative psychological energy.

In a strict sense, however, most of these techniques are not ergogenic aids. Many are *psychotherapeutic techniques*. Others are actually a form of mental training, as already discussed, and, like physical training, take time to develop before showing any benefits. However, since many of these techniques have not been applied extensively to sport, sport psychologists often refer to them as ergogenic aids when they are used in attempts to improve performance. When applied to improve athletic performance these methods have also been called *psychodoping* (but this term is not common).

Elite athletes and those involved in sports with complex skill require ments usually need assistance in order to realize their full athletic potentials. In most cases their physical-training program is individualized and their skill development is refined under the watchful eye of a knowledgeable coach and trainer. Any medical problems they develop are treated promptly by appropriate sports medicine personnel. On the other hand, some athletes in sports at lower levels of competition or in sports involving simple skills may design, initiate, and refine their own physical-training programs and treat their minor injuries themselves. For example, thousands of the athletes participating in mass sporting events, such as marathons and triathlons, have developed their own programs and trained themselves.

A similar situation exists with mental training. Some athletes may need the assistance of a trained professional if they have complex psychological needs. Just as athletes with serious medical problems need the care of a physician, the psychologically disturbed athlete needs the counsel of a clinical psychologist. Clinical sport psychologists can assess psychopathological conditions in athletes and provide appropriate psychotherapy. They may help athletes with drug-dependency problems and various eating disorders, such as *anorexia nervosa* and *bulimia*. Fortunately, most of the psychological problems that lead to performance decrements in sport are not pathological in nature; they can be treated by professionals other than clinical psychologists or even by the athletes themselves.

Educational sport psychologists may be compared to the coach or trainer. They may help the athlete reach his or her psychological potential through the use of proper mental-training techniques, such as many of those listed in Table 6.1. In a sense, these techniques may be regarded as ergogenic aids. Although many of the techniques listed in Table 6.1, such as *hypnosis*, are best applied under the control of a trained sport psychologist, some may be learned and applied by other professionals, such as coaches.

Also, several of the psychological ergogenic aids listed in Table 6.1 are self-applicable, so athletes may learn a few techniques and develop their own mental-training programs. One of the leading sport psychologists in the United States indicates that self-application is probably the most practical approach to the use of psychological ergogenic aids, for then athletes may control their own psychological energy levels before and during competition. They also have the advantage of knowing that they are in control of their psychological energy and do not have to rely on another individual.

The remainder of this chapter will focus on several of the simple psychological ergogenic aids that you can learn and use under appropriate circumstances. They are grouped into two basic categories. *Psychological energizers* are designed to elevate your psychological energy or to maximize your positive psychological energy. *Psychological tranquilizers* are designed to reduce disruptive psychological energy or to minimize your negative psychological energy. Although the discussion of these aids will be separated, it is important to note that athletes often use both types of aids together. Depending on the technique, the aid may be designed to serve as a psychological energizer or tranquilizer.

Psychological Energizers

Theoretical Basis

A song that was once popular in this country contains the lyrics, "You gotta accentuate the positive, eliminate the negative, and don't mess with Mister In-Between." These lyrics underlie the basic theoretical value of psychological energizers as a means of improving athletic performance. You have to accentuate those techniques that maximize your positive psychological energy and eliminate those factors that generate negative psychological energy. In a sense, psychological energizers are comparable to the pharmacological stimulants discussed in chapter 4. They are designed to stimulate you naturally by mobilizing your own natural sources of stimulant hormones.

Psychological energizers may be useful when you are on the left side of the inverted U continuum and in a state of low arousal. You may be there for a variety of reasons. For example, you may be bored because your level of ability is so much greater than the demands of the task confronting you. Conversely, you may have a low level of self-confidence because the task is well beyond your ability and your negative thoughts may lead to a state of depression.

A low arousal state will affect your performance both in practice and in competition. One of the most important aspects underlying your motivation to train hard in practice is the specific goal that you have set for yourself. If you have no goal in mind, your motivation level, which is actually your state of arousal, will most likely be low. Failure to train properly in practice usually translates to failure in competition. In addition, a low arousal state in competition due to boredom or overconfidence will most likely lead

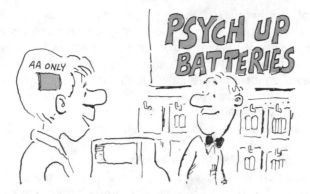

"I need a couple of double AAs to psych myself up."

to poor concentration in the task at hand. In such cases you are more likely to be distracted by external factors, such as the jeering of the crowd when you are attempting a free throw.

The basic theory underlying the use of psychological energizers to improve athletic performance is to stimulate you to your optimal arousal zone. In some cases you may need to increase your positive psychological energy beyond your normal level of arousal; at other times you may need to restore your normal levels that have been depressed by negative psychological energy sources. In this regard, sport psychologists have applied a variety of techniques to sport, including most of those listed in Table 6.1. Among the more popular techniques are *goal setting, attentional skill training, thought control,* and *imagery.* Goal-setting techniques are designed to increase motivation for practice. Attentional skill training helps the athlete to concentrate. Thought control attempts to eliminate negative thoughts and emphasize positive ones. Imagery techniques are designed to create positive mental images of performance. Often several of these techniques are used together.

Research Findings

Although sport psychology is one of the youngest of the sports sciences in terms of research, a substantial number of studies have been conducted over the past 20 years relative to the use of various psychological energizers. Much of the research has focused on the effectiveness of imagery and related techniques, such as *mental rehearsal, covert rehearsal strategies,* and *visual motor behavioral rehearsal* (VMBR). The use of *posthypnotic suggestions* to induce an ergogenic effect has also received considerable research attention.

Several prominent sport psychologists, including Rod Dishman, Dan Landers, Rainer Martens, William P. Morgan, and John Silva, have conducted extensive reviews of the research in this area. In general they note that although the theory underlying the use of psychological energizers to improve performance in sport is sound, the research evidence available at this time is not conclusive, particulary when applied to elite athletes. Nevertheless, they do note that the evidence is somewhat supportive and offer a cautious endorsement, suggesting that the use of psychological aids may be better than no treatment at all. Moreover, they suggest that the application of psychological aids to athletes be individualized, for a technique that benefits some might prove detrimental to others. This finding has recently been supported by several studies from Dr. Morgan's Sport Psychology Laboratory at the University of Wisconsin.

Survey research with athletes has revealed that many of them are currently using various psychological energizers before and during competition. Among the most popular are several to be discussed here, including thought control and imagery.

Recommendations

You may have low levels of psychological energy for a number of reasons. One may be that you are simply tired physically. Participating in sports demands physical energy; if your physical energy sources are low you will also suffer psychologically. Therefore, you must attend to the basics of adequate sleep and rest and proper nutrition. Another reason may be your lack of confidence to perform at a level necessary for success. If your lack of confidence is related to inadequate physical training, then again you need to get back to the basics—in this case proper training to improve your fitness and skill levels.

If you are physically well prepared for competition but aware that low-arousal levels may be hampering your performance, you may wish to consider the application of one or more psychological energizers. Research has suggested that they may be helpful, particularly when individualized and self-administered. As they appear to be harmless for most healthy athletes, there do not seem to be any legal, ethical, or medical problems associated with their use to improve performance. However, because these techniques are most useful when individualized, it is important that you are aware of your own special needs so that you may plan appropriate actions. It is also important to note that many of these techniques are forms of mental training and, just like physical training, may require much practice before maximal benefits are realized.

The scope of this book does not permit a detailed discussion of the various psychological energizers that may be applied to sport. If you are interested in an expanded coverage, you may wish to consult one or more of the excellent textbooks listed in the reference section. The books by Martens, Nideffer, Orlick, and Suinn are very practical. The following limited discussion will focus on the essence of four techniques that you may try: goal setting, imagery, attention training, and thought control.

Goal Setting.   Although goal setting may not seem like an ergogenic aid, it may help you psychologically by providing the internal motivation to train harder in practice and perform better in competition. In sports, your ultimate objective should be excellence, to be all that you can possibly be. It is the drive towards excellence that will sustain your motivation and dedication to improve. Unfortunately, most of us in sports do not actually know how good we can be, so we establish performance goals in pursuit of our concept of excellence. These goals can serve as psychological energizers.

The performance goals you establish in pursuit of excellence will depend on the sport. But there are certain characteristics of goal setting applicable to all sports. First, in terms of time to accomplish them, goals may be characterized as either *long-range* or *short-range*. Second, the athlete should possess the physical abilities to attain these goals, so they must be realistic. Third, the goal must be specific in nature, such as a 4-minute mile or a 7-foot high jump. Finally, a number of manageable short-term goals should be developed in pursuit of the long-range goal.

To help illustrate these points, let me relate a story to you about a friend of mine who wanted to qualify to run the Boston Marathon. At the time, his standard for qualification was to run another marathon in 3 hours or less. He had been into running for about a year, averaging about 45 minutes to run a 10-kilometer road race. I explained to him that a marathon is 42.2 kilometers, or more than four 10-kilometer races, so even if he was able to maintain his current 10-kilometer pace for the full marathon his time would still be over 3 hours. In his current state of fitness, his goal of a 3-hour

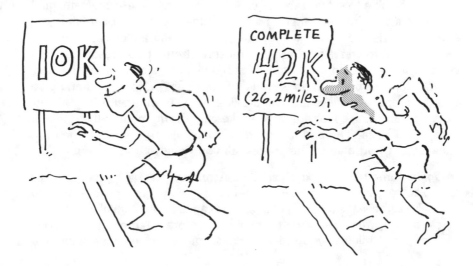

marathon was not realistic. However, perusal of his training program showed some definite room for improvement, for he was averaging less than 15 miles per week, mostly slow distance work. He could also afford to lose about 15 pounds of body fat.

One of the first things I did was to pace him around our quarter-mile track in a time of 1:43. Although he was breathing hard, he experienced no extreme discomfort. But he was clearly over his anaerobic threshold and relying somewhat on his lactic acid energy system. When I indicated to him that he needed to run about 105 consecutive quartermiles at that pace in order to run a marathon in 3 hours, he realized the enormity of the task confronting him. However, as he was highly motivated, we established the 3-hour marathon as a long-range goal. Given the room he had for improvement, it appeared realistic.

His training program was redesigned by gradually increasing his total weekly mileage and eventually incorporating speed work through interval training. Although he participated in a variety of races, we focused on his 10-kilometer times as short-term goals for improvement. Based on predictive formulas, a 10-kilometer time of 38:30 should provide him with the speed and reserve to complete a 3-hour marathon provided he also had adequate mileage in his training. Over a 3-year period we continued to modify his short-term goals as he ran faster times in the 10-kilometer. Another short-term goal was simply completing a full marathon, without being concerned with the time, which he did twice. It took him 3 years, but he eventually broke 39 minutes in the 10-kilometer and completed the marathon in just under 3 hours to qualify for Boston.

For my friend the long-range goal was realistic and specific. The short-term goals established were also specific and manageable in reasonable amounts of time. Depending on your level of expertise in a given sport you may be able to set your own goals, but in many cases successful goal setting requires the assistance of a knowledgeable coach or trainer.

As a final note on goal setting, the goal for many athletes is simply to win. To want to win is fine, but you must realize that you really have no control over the outcome of any athletic contest. You cannot control your competition. All you can do is focus on your own performance and give your best; proper goal setting can provide you with the means to do your best. To paraphrase Gandhi, if you take care of the means, the end will take care of itself. The end may or may not be victory, but it will be pure excellence if you give to the contest all you have to give.

Imagery.   Imagery can be a very successful psychological energizer, for it may be used in a variety of ways and for a variety of purposes. Imagery can help set the stage for competition. You can use it to get highly aroused, or psyched-up, as a weight lifter might do before attempting a lift. You can use it to familiarize yourself with a race course, as an alpine skier may do for a downhill run. You can use it to perfect your skill just prior to execution, as a high jumper might mentally rehearse the approach, takeoff, clearance, and landing. You can use it during competition to energize yourself as you recall the feeling you had during one of your previous peak performances. Imagery may also be an integral part of other psychological energizers, such as thought control.

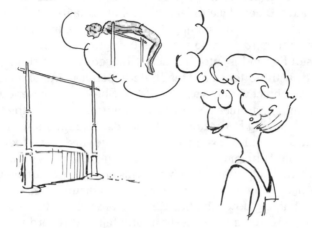

Several aids exist that may be used along with imagery during training. Musical tapes, such as the themes from *Chariots of Fire*, or *Rocky*, may stimulate images of training along the beach in slow motion or charging up a hill like a powerful machine. Videotapes of highly skilled performances, either one of your own peak performances or one of an elite athlete (such as used in Sybervision), may help you form a mental image of perfect form. However, for use in competition, the most practical technique is to develop your own mental images for specific purposes in your sport.

Imagery is often referred to as *the mind's eye*, but it can be more than that. It can be used to mentally experience all of your senses. Your eyes and ears capture visual and auditory stimuli to be conducted to your brain, but it is your brain, or mind, that sees and hears. In using imagery you should attempt to recall all appropriate sensations, particularly seeing, hearing, feeling, and, if relevant, smelling and tasting.

When first learning imagery you should select a quiet environment free from distractions and be completely relaxed. You might want to use one of the techniques discussed in the psychological tranquilizer section to achieve a state of relaxation with your eyes closed. You may initially try out all five senses. Focus in on this morning. Can you see yourself dressing? Can you see it in color? Can you hear the birds sing, the toaster pop, the door shut? Can you feel the texture of the clothes you put on? Can you smell the coffee or burnt toast? Can you taste the strawberry preserves on your toast? These may not be appropriate examples for you, but try to imagine some specific aspects of your morning environment that will trigger your five senses, and then attempt to recreate them mentally.

As there are a variety of applications of imagery to sport, so the images you create will be specific to the particular outcome you desire. The mental images you create are limited only by your imagination. As a brief example, let us consider a runner preparing for a mile race. In preparation she might find a quiet place to lean back and visualize herself as relaxed, alert, and confident at the starting line. She focuses upon her own inner strength and the hard training that has brought her here. She hears the starter's pistol fire and is into the race. She sees herself running smooth and relaxed, with no tension. Her stride is perfect, and she can feel her shoe making contact with the track surface. She can hear her own breathing, relaxed and rhythmical. She visualizes herself breaking the tape at the finish and celebrating her victory with friends. She may also use imagery during the race itself. For example, she may see, hear, and feel a big wind at her back that is helping to push her along. She may visualize herself as a well-oiled, finely tuned machine cruising along effortlessly. Finally, as she approaches the finishing stretch she can picture herself as a driving locomotive charging down the track. Afterwards, if she has won, she may use imagery to recreate the sensations she felt and record these for later use during training sessions. If she lost she may mentally rehearse any possible errors and attempt to eliminate them through proper practice.

The images you create will be specific to your sport, but in order to use them in competition you need to develop them in practice. Apply them while you are training, as they may allow you to train more effectively and may benefit your competitive performance. You also need to practice them in simulated competitive situations, such as before a crowd.

Imagery is based on the power of suggestion, the ability to create positive images that may help increase your positive psychological energy. In order to maximize the effectiveness of imagery you need to believe in the image and expect it to happen. Imagery is not magic, but it can help.

Attention Training.   Attention training is basically just that—training athletes to improve their focus of attention. Despite the small distinction between attention and concentration the terms are often used interchangeably, and some sport psychologists prefer the term *concentration training*. In essence, concentration is simply a more narrow form of attention. Because our discussion here is brief, we will not distinguish between the two terms.

Attention is the energy we devote to receiving cues from our environment and interpreting them for possible action. Robert Nideffer, an internationally renowned sport psychologist, has noted that athletes need to respond to both internal and external cues. The internal cues come from within the body, whereas the external cues come from the surrounding environment. The athlete may also have to respond to a varying number of cues, sometimes only one but at other times many.

As is probably obvious then, the degree of attention or concentration needed by an athlete in competition depends on the sport. A classic example is the different attention needs of a golfer and of a quarterback in professional football. During putting, the center of attention for the golfer is on applying just the right amount of force to that little white ball staring at him. Cues from the external environment are few. In contrast, the quarterback coming out of the huddle and approaching the line has a myriad of external cues deserving his attention. He must analyze the opponent's defense in order to change the play if necessary and must know the pass routes for all of his receivers.

The degree of attention may also change during different stages of the sport. Between pitches, a shortstop in baseball may let his mind wander, scan the crowd, think about what he is going to do after the game, or whatever. However, with runners on first and second base and the pitcher ready to deliver, he needs to focus his attention sharply on the actions he will take if and when the hitter hits the ball. If he misses any cues, he may end up a step behind.

As you continue to learn the nature of your sport you will likely pick up those cues that are important and deserving of your attention or concentration. However, a number of factors may lead to a loss of concentration during sport. Boredom, distraction by the crowd, excessive stress, negative thoughts, being psyched-out by an opponent, and physical fatigue

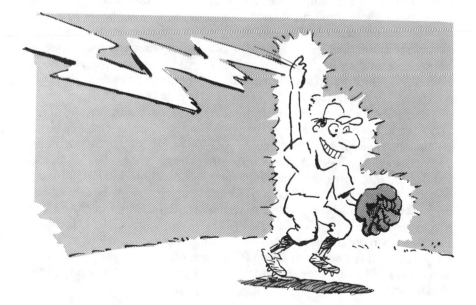

can all cause the mind to drift. Attention training is designed to prevent or minimize the effect of these factors on your concentration level during sport.

Attention training is designed to provide you cues that help you focus your attention and concentrate on the task at hand. You will need to develop techniques specific to the concentration demands of your sport. One technique is to develop a set of rituals that remind you to concentrate; these rituals might involve other psychological energizers, like imagery. For example, in the situation just described the shortstop might raise his arm overhead as a ritual trigger to focus his attention. At the same time he might visualize a bolt of lightning entering his body to energize him for action. As will be discussed shortly, thought-control techniques can also help to focus attention. As with any other psychological ergogenic aid, you will need to develop your own strategies and practice them constantly.

Thought Control.   Underlying thought control as a psychological energizer is the basic premise that if you do not control your thoughts, they will control you. You talk to yourself many times throughout the day, and this self-talk is nothing more than a series of thoughts, some of them positive and some of them negative. As applied to sport, thought-control techniques are designed to maximize your positive thoughts and minimize or eliminate your negative ones. The latter objective may be more important, for *although research has shown that positive thoughts do not always increase performance, negative thoughts almost always decrease it.*

Negative thoughts appear in athletes for a variety of reasons, but those relevant to sports are usually due to low levels of self-confidence in regard to the competition or performance at hand. In order to eliminate negative thoughts during sport you have to recognize that they exist. A good idea is simply to count over several days the number of times you feel negative thoughts about your performance ability. Carry a pad with you and write them down. Once you have identified those that may be exerting a negative impact, you can design a program to eliminate them. The goal is not only to eliminate negative thoughts, but to replace them with positive ones.

The key to preventing negative thoughts is to stop them just as they begin to develop. Treat negative thoughts as you are encouraged to treat a friend who offers you drugs—just say *NO*. Another choice word is *STOP*. In this manner you may consciously eliminate negative thoughts. Initially you may wish to actually say out loud *NO* or *STOP*, although this might be embarrassing in some circumstances. You may also say *STOP* mentally and use imagery to create a picture of a huge red stop sign in your mind. Imagery may be used in other ways to remove negative thoughts, such as touching the ground and visualizing the thought flowing out of your body. Try these approaches. The next time you hear yourself saying *I can't*, get rid of that thought immediately.

Replace negative thoughts with positive thoughts. One approach is to use a positive word or phrase appropriate for your sport that may help to energize you, such as GO, DRIVE, PUSH, or MOVE IT. If you need to increase your attention, such words may also be part of your ritual before or during competition to remind you to concentrate. Also, imagery can enhance the effectiveness of these positive thoughts. For example, as you are becoming fatigued use these energizing words in conjunction with an image of one of your peak performances. You may not be able to leap tall buildings in a single bound, but such techniques can provide you with that additional amount of energy you need. Learn to say *I can*.

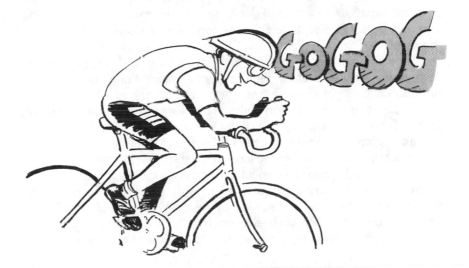

Psychological Tranquilizers

Theoretical Basis

If you review the inverted U theory illustrated in Figure 6.3 you will see that too much psychological energy may actually become a negative force. Psychological arousal beyond the optimal zone may harm performance. At this point you might begin to experience some of the symptoms of anxiety or excessive stress.

The Stress Response.   Through the process of evolution your body has developed a series of reactions in response to physical threats to your safety. For the caveman the threat might have been a confrontation with a saber-toothed tiger. For you the threat might be the sudden approach of a growling dog while you are jogging. Your mind quickly evaluates the danger and your body immediately responds with a series of physiological reactions, such as increased blood flow, increased oxygen uptake, and increased muscle activity, that heightens your ability for energy production to counteract this threat to your safety. Once you are safe you are amazed at how fast you climbed that tree. What you have experienced is known as the *stress response*.

Your thoughts alone can also trigger the stress response. Simply thinking about the growling dog can initiate the same physiological responses, as well as some psychological and behavioral responses. In this example, your thoughts perceive a threat to your physical safety. But you may also perceive threats to your mental safety, or to your reputation. For example, you may be a superior athlete whose confident performance has earned the respect of thousands of fans. But for some reason you have developed a fear of public speaking. If you believe a poor speaking performance can damage your reputation, then simply the thought of addressing a class of 20 students might elicit the stress response. Your body does not distinguish whether your perception of threat involves physical safety or mental safety. Table 6.2 presents some of the possible physiological, psychological, and behavioral consequences of the stress response.

Physical threats to your safety exist in most sports. In some sports, such as sky diving and mountain climbing, athletes accept the challenge of very serious threats. In almost all sports there is the chance of some physical injury, such as the prevalence of knee injuries in American football. If you are a 150-pound novice linebacker confronted head-on by a 250-pound charging fullback you may perceive possible physical trauma and experi-

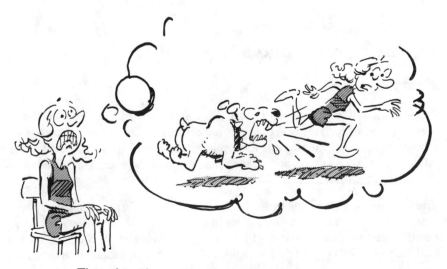

Thoughts alone may trigger the stress response.

TABLE 6.2
POSSIBLE CONSEQUENCES OF THE STRESS RESPONSE

PHYSIOLOGICAL

Increased heart rate	Increased blood flow to muscles
Increased blood pressure	Increased oxygen uptake
Increased breathing rate	Increased sweating
Increased blood glucose	Increased secretion of adrenalin
Decreased salivation	

PSYCHOLOGICAL

Decreased mental flexibility	Decreased ability to focus on the external environment
Decreased decision-making ability	
Decreased ability to concentrate	Increased focus on personal feelings
Increased number of negative thoughts	

BEHAVIORAL

Increased muscle twitching and trembling	Increased tendency to rush things
	Decreased voice control
Increased speed of talking	

ence the stress response. In general, however, experienced athletes learn to suppress thoughts of physical harm during competition.

Mental threats to your physical safety also exist in sports. Simply thinking about possible physical harm may trigger the stress response, such as a skydiver who contemplates parachute failure just as he or she is about to exit the plane at 10,000 feet. However, the most common mental threat perceived by athletes is probably the fear of failure to live up to performance expectations, either their own expectations or those of others, such as coaches or parents.

As is probably obvious by now, the physiological, psychological, and behavioral responses to excess anxiety or stress may interfere with optimal athletic performance. Physiologically, a more rapid heart rate allows less time for a pistol shooter to fire between beats. Psychologically, negative thoughts and lack of concentration impair performance in a wide variety of events. Behaviorally, muscle tension that results in trembling and twitching interferes with optimal aiming in sports such as riflery and archery.

The stress response occurs in all levels of sport, from Little League to professional. Although it may occur in a few athletes in almost every contest, stress usually occurs when there is an increased importance associated with an event, such as a championship at stake. In such situations arousal level is increased excessively and the resultant state of anxiety often affects performance. This state of anxiety in sport has been expressed in a variety of ways; we have all heard of athletes who have "choked" or been "psyched-out."

Stress Reduction.   Psychological tranquilizers are theorized to reduce levels of anxiety, or psychological arousal, and help the athlete reach the optimal arousal zone. In their use in attempts to prevent adverse effects of the stress response, they may be compared to pharmacological depressants. For example, you may recall from chapter 4 that pistol shooters have used beta-blockers to slow the heart rate and reduce muscle trembling.

Psychological techniques to reduce anxiety have usually been classified under the general term of *stress management*. As applied to sport, psychological tranquilizers are designed to decrease disruptive stress that may interfere with optimal performance. They may be used to induce relaxation for proper rest and recovery on a day-to-day basis, but in competition they are designed to help the athlete be relaxed yet alert.

Research Findings

Stress-management techniques have been used for medical or psychotherapeutic purposes for a number of years. *Biofeedback, progressive muscular relaxation, relaxation imagery, auditory and visual relaxation tapes, flotation tanks*, and other methods, even aerobic exercise programs, have been used with patients in attempts to reduce blood pressure, neuromuscular tension, and psychological stress. Both clinical and experimental evidence suggest that such techniques may be helpful adjuncts to other therapeutic procedures in medicine.

According to one prominent sport psychologist, research efforts to evaluate the ergogenic effectiveness of stress-management techniques are still in the infancy stage. Although a considerable number of studies have been conducted, many of the earlier experimental designs have been seriously challenged because of faulty protocols. For our purposes here there is no need to review individual research studies, for several major reviews of the available scientific research have recently been written by some of the most respected sport psychologists in the United States. In general, they have noted that the data supporting an ergogenic effect of stress-management procedures as a means of improving physical performance are not very convincing.

On the other hand, they also note that the theoretical basis is sound. As with psychological energizers, the use of psychological tranquilizers by athletes may be better than no treatment at all. As one sport psychologist noted, some of the research showing beneficial results of stress-management procedures should be interpreted as what *can* happen, not what *will* happen. Thus, the application of some of the procedures about to be discussed may be helpful to you if they help reduce excess anxiety and return you to your personal optimal arousal zone.

Recommendations

If you recognize that certain sports situations evoke a stress response in you, such as a pounding heart, nervous tension, sweating, negative thoughts, and the inability to concentrate, then you may be a candidate for stress-management procedures. One of the first things you want to do is determine the cause of the stress response. *In many situations stress is a result of low self-confidence or fear of failure.* Low self-confidence can trigger a vicious cycle of negative thoughts, high anxiety levels, disturbance of mental and physical functions, and poor performance, the latter reinforcing your feelings of low self-confidence. If low self-confidence and fear of failure contribute to your state of anxiety, you may wish to review the section on goal setting and the emphasis placed on winning presented earlier in this chapter. If you establish realistic goals and give all you have to attain them, you should not expect anything more from yourself. There is considerable wisdom in the old adage that it is not whether you win or lose, but how you play the game.

Many times in sport the pressure appears greater than normal. The pressure on you as the leadoff batter in the first inning of a regular season game appears far less than the pressure involved in being at the plate with two outs in the bottom of the ninth, the bases loaded, and your team down by one run in the championship game. You can probably think of a number of such situations in your sport. If you experience the stress response under such conditions, use of stress-management techniques may be helpful to you.

Four different strategies for coping with stress will be presented, although you will see similarities among them. They will be covered only briefly, but you will be given enough information to practice them if you so desire. The first strategy involves breathing exercises and is also used as a preliminary to the other three techniques, namely meditation, relaxation imagery, and autogenic relaxation training.

Deep Breathing.   Deep breathing may be an effective means of reducing stress. Take a deep breath, as deep as you can, hold it for a few seconds, then let it out slowly. Do you feel a little sense of relaxation? In essence, a breathing exercise for relaxation should involve slow, deep inhalation and prolonged exhalation. The exercise is primarily useful prior to performance, but may be used as a key to relax and concentrate during performance. The following represents one approach.

1. Assume a comfortable position, either sitting relaxed in a chair or, preferably, lying down on your back, eyes closed, and muscles relaxed.
2. Inhale slowly and deeply through the nose only (though you may use the mouth if nose breathing is uncomfortable). As you inhale, slowly count in your mind from one to five so that you do not rush your breathing. Feel your chest and stomach expand as you continue to inhale. Focus your mind on the act of inhalation.
3. Once you have reached a state of full inhalation, hold that position for 3 to 5 seconds and think to yourself, *I am very calm and relaxed.*
4. Exhale slowly through both the mouth and the nose. As you do, count down mentally from five to one. Concentrate on exhaling as much air as possible. If you are alone, an alternate approach is to close your mouth and emit the sound *om*. Say a long *ooooommmmmmm*, concentrating on the sound and the gentle vibrations in your head.

Meditation.   Meditation is a relaxation technique derived from Eastern religious customs. It became popular in the United States in the 1960s in a form known as *transcendental meditation*, or *TM*. In TM, each individual has a *mantra*, which is a particular sound or word used during the meditation session. The following guidelines may be used to practice meditation.

1. Find a quiet area and sit quietly with your eyes closed. Do several breathing exercises to relax. Think about relaxing your whole body.
2. Choose a mantra that has little significance to you, such as *om* or the number one. Associate the mantra with your breathing, mentally picturing the word *om* or the number one as you inhale and exhale. Do not think about, feel, or visualize anything but your mantra. Repeat it over and over again in your mind. Do not let any other thoughts distract you. Always return to your mantra.
3. After about 20 to 30 minutes, or less time if necessary, open your eyes and sit quietly for several minutes while you phase out your mantra. Then make a strong fist with each hand and say to yourself, "I am totally awake and alert, but relaxed and refreshed."

Relaxation Imagery.   Relaxation imagery is a form of meditation, but instead of thinking of a mantra you visualize a relaxing scene. The principles of relaxation imagery are comparable to those discussed under the section on psychological energizers. Relaxation imagery often precedes the use of other forms of psychological energizers (prior to athletic competition). To practice relaxation imagery simply follow the steps for meditation above, but substitute your mantra with an appropriate image. Helpful images usually convey feelings of warmth, heaviness, or floating, such as riding on a magic carpet in a warm wind or sinking into a soft cloud and being warmed by the sun.

Relaxation imagery.

Autogenic Relaxation Training.   Autogenic relaxation training is a form of self-hypnosis designed to produce specific body sensations associated with relaxation. Feelings of warmth and heaviness are stressed. A description of a basic autogenic relaxation technique follows. Although you can make the suggestions in step 3 to yourself, it may be a good idea to tape them for playback to simplify the process.

1. Find a quiet place to relax, assume a comfortable lying or sitting position, and close your eyes. Do several repetitions of the breathing exercises to induce relaxation.
2. Remove all possible distractions and repeat to yourself three times, "I am totally relaxed and feel good about myself."
3. Starting from your head and working down to your toes, progressively relax parts of your body by creating sensations of warmth or

heaviness. Slowly repeat in your mind each of the following phrases three times; as you do, try to visualize the warmth or heaviness.

My head and neck feel heavy.

My shoulders feel heavy.

My right arm feels heavy.

My left arm feels heavy.

My chest feels heavy.

My stomach feels heavy.

My right leg feels heavy.

My left leg feels heavy.

My head and neck feel warm and calm.

My shoulders feel warm and calm.

My right arm feels warm and calm.

My left arm feels warm and calm.

My chest feels warm and calm.

My stomach feels warm and calm.

My right leg feels warm and calm.

My left leg feels warm and calm.

My breathing is calm.

My heart rate is calm.

I am totally relaxed and feel good about myself.

4. When finished, open your eyes and say to yourself "I am totally awake and alert, but relaxed and refreshed."

A modification of the autogenic relaxation technique is *progressive muscular relaxation*. Basically, you use the same sequence as just described for the various body parts, but you also induce a strong isometric muscle contraction, hold it for several seconds, then release it slowly while repeating the heavy and warm phrases.

To maximize the possible benefits derived from these psychological tranquilizers, they must be practiced. Once you learn to do them in the quiet of your room, you may be able to use them just prior to athletic competition. In some cases you might be able to find a quiet spot, but you can also learn to use these techniques with people milling about. Just lie back and focus on your mantra. If you feel yourself getting tight in competition you may use the breathing exercise as a cue (and as a means) to relax, possibly also saying *relax* to yourself as a key positive word to help focus your concentration.

For those interested, more detailed coverage of stress-management procedures can be found in a variety of other texts, including *Guide to Stress Reduction* by L. John Mason, *The Relaxation Response* by Herbert Benson, *Progressive Relaxation* by Edmund Jacobson, and *Controlling Stress and Tension* by D. Girdano and G. Everly. Other sport-psychology texts mentioned previously, such as the ones by Martens and Suinn, contain a chapter on stress-management strategies.

As a final point for this chapter, it is important to know that your relationships with others around you, such as parents, coaches, friends and teammates, can have a significant impact on your performance in sports. Consequently, the elimination of negative thoughts and the incorporation of positive thoughts in areas of your life outside sports is an important objective. With this in mind we present the Optimist's Creed.

THE OPTIMIST'S CREED

Promise Yourself

To be so strong that nothing can disturb your peace of mind.

To talk health, happiness and prosperity to every person you meet.

To make all your friends feel there is something in them.

To look at the sunny side of everything and make your optimism come true.

To think only of the best, to work only for the best and expect only the best.

To be just as enthusiastic about the success of others as you are about your own.

To forget the mistakes of the past and press on to the greater achievements of the future.

To wear a cheerful countenance at all times and give every living creature you meet a smile.

To give so much time to the improvement of yourself that you have no time to criticize others.

To be too large for worry, too noble for anger, too strong for fear, and too happy to permit the presence of trouble.

Optimist International

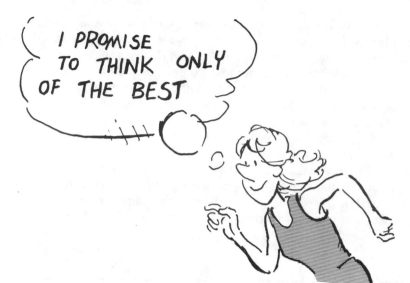

Selected Readings

Books

Benson, H. (1975). *The relaxation response.* New York: William Morrow.

Girdano, D., & Everly, G. (1979). *Controlling stress and tension.* Englewood Cliffs, NJ: Prentice Hall.

Jacobson, E. (1974). *Progressive relaxation.* Chicago: University of Chicago Press.

Kubistant, T. (1986). *Performing your best: A guide to psychological skills for high achievers.* Champaign, IL: Life Enhancement.

Martens, R. (1987). *Coaches guide to sport psychology.* Champaign, IL: Human Kinetics.

Mason, L. (1980). *Guide to stress reduction.* Culver City, CA: Peace Press.

Nideffer, R. (1985). *Athlete's guide to mental training.* Champaign, IL: Human Kinetics.

Nideffer, R., & Sharpe, R. (1978). *Attention control training.* New York: Wyden Books.

Orlick, T. (1986). *Psyching for sport.* Champaign, IL: Leisure Press.

Silva, J., & Weinberg, R. (1984). *Psychological foundations of sport.* Champaign, IL: Human Kinetics.

Singer, R. (1986). *Peak performance . . . and more.* Ithaca, NY: Mouvement Publications.

Suinn, R. (1986). *Seven steps to peak performance.* Toronto: Han Huber.
Vanek, M., & Cratty, B. (1970). *Psychology and the superior athlete.* London: Macmillan.

Reviews

Coker, E. (1987). Improved strength performance through goal setting. *National Strength and Conditioning Association Journal,* **9**(3), 48-49.
Dishman, R. (1983). Stress management procedures. In M. Williams, (Ed.), *Ergogenic aids in sport* (pp. 275-320). Champaign, IL: Human Kinetics.
Finn, J. (1985). Competitive excellence: It's a matter of mind and body. *The Physician and Sportsmedicine,* **13**(2), 61-75.
Hatfield, B., & Landers, D. (1987). Psychophysiology in exercise and sport research: An overview. *Exercise and Sport Sciences Reviews,* **15**, 351-387.
Hatfield, B., & Walford, G. (1987). Understanding anxiety: Implications for sport performance. *National Strength and Conditioning Association Journal,* **9**(2), 58-65.
Krenz, E. (1986). Hypnosis versus autogenic training: A comparison. *American Journal of Clinical Hypnosis,* **28**, 209-213.
Morgan, W. (1985). Psychogenic factors and exercise metabolism: A review. *Medicine and Science in Sports and Exercise,* **17**, 309-316.
Morgan, W., & Brown, D. (1983). Hypnosis. In M. Williams (Ed.), *Ergogenic aids in sport* (pp. 223-252). Champaign, IL: Human Kinetics.
Nideffer, R. (1987). Psychological preparation of the highly competitive athlete. *The Physician and Sportsmedicine,* **15**(10), 85-94.
Silva, J. (1983). Covert rehearsal strategies. In M. Williams (Ed.), *Ergogenic aids in sport* (pp. 253-274). Champaign, IL: Human Kinetics.
Ziegler, S. (1987). Negative thought stopping: A key to performance enhancement. *Journal of Physical Education, Recreation and Dance,* **58**(4), 66-69.

Chapter 7

Mechanical
and Biomechanical
Ergogenic Aids

MECHANICS IS DEFINED AS THE SCIENCE of force and matter. It is
the study of stationary and moving objects (matter) and the forces that cause
them to move or to remain stationary. When this science is applied to the
study of humans and other living beings it is known as *biomechanics*.
Furthermore, a subspecialty area of biomechanics is *sports biomechanics*,
which involves the application of mechanical and biomechanical principles
to the study of movement in sport.

All sports involve the movement of matter. In some sports the main object to move is the body itself, which is a collection of different forms of
matter such as bones, muscles, and fat. Running and high jumping are
examples of two sports in which we are primarily interested in moving our
bodies as fast or as high as we can. However, we are also moving other
matter in these two sports, such as the shoes and the uniform being worn.

In other sports our primary goal is to move matter other than our bodies
with optimal speed, distance, or accuracy. A wide variety of external objects are used in sports and each has its own characteristics in the amount,
type, and design of matter. Just think of the dozens of different types of
balls used for such sports as baseball, basketball, football, tennis, golf, soccer,
field hockey, jai alai, as well as the objects used in other sports, such as
the javelin, shot, discus, hammer, arrow, and bullet. Although we may
give movement directly to many of these objects, we often need to move
or control another object that imparts the force for movement, such as a
baseball bat, tennis racket, golf club, bow, or rifle. In still other sports the
athlete needs to control an object that is the basis for participation, such
as a bicycle, bobsled, or sailboat.

Forces are able to produce or stop motion. In chapter 2 we learned that the three human energy systems are designed to convert *chemical energy* into *mechanical energy*, resulting in force production through the mechanics of muscular contraction. In the preceding four chapters we have discussed the possible roles of nutritional, pharmacological, physiological, and psychological ergogenic aids as means of regulating force production through the optimal use of human energy. For many sports we were interested in ways to maximize energy production and force development that would improve performance, such as the use of blood doping by endurance athletes or anabolic steroids by weight lifters. In other sports, however, we were interested in reducing excessive muscle tension and tremor that could disrupt optimal performance, by the use of certain psychological techniques with archers, for example. In general then, within the limitations of our genetic background, our state of training, and the effectiveness of the ergogenic aids we have mentioned, we are able to control muscular force production through regulation of the three human energy systems. We can use this energy to generate force to either produce or stop motion.

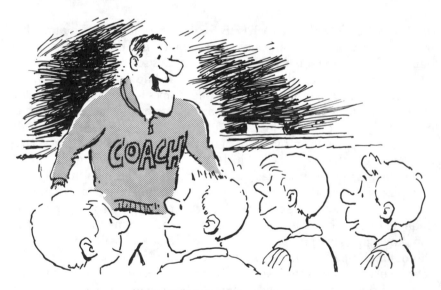

"May the force be with you."

In all sports somebody or something provides *resistance* to our goal. The basic nature of sport would not exist without competition, so in a sense our opponents always provide a form of resistance. In some events resistance provided by an opponent is not physical in nature, such as swimming and running in separate lanes, as there is no actual physical contact. On the other hand, our opponents can provide considerable physical resistance in such sports as wrestling and judo.

Natural Forces

Of interest to us from the viewpoint of the application of mechanical ergogenic aids to sport is the physical resistance to athletic performance provided by nature. In many sports we use our *internal forces* generated through muscle contraction to overcome some of the *external forces* in nature that resist movement. Although a variety of external forces exist in nature, the ones that have the most significant effect on athletic performance are *gravitational force, frictional force,* and *forces found in moving fluids* (both air and water are considered fluids by the physicist).

In some sports these forces may actually help to improve performance. An obvious example would be riding a bicycle downhill, where the pulling force of gravity aids acceleration. Fluid forces such as a wind at the back of a cyclist or runner or a following current for a triathlete in the swim portion of competition will also provide an additional forward force to increase speed. In some sports these forces are the basis for moving the athlete. Skydivers and downhill skiers depend on gravity to provide motion, whereas sailors rely on wind and surfers on waves of water.

Usually, though, external forces provide resistance to movement in sport. Athletes who attempt to jump to great heights, such as high jumpers and pole vaulters, are basically fighting the force of gravity. Downhill skiers face increased air resistance, whereas sprint swimmers experience high levels of water resistance. Increased frictional forces, such as the increased resistance of wet snow for a cross-country skier, may also impede performance.

The basic purpose of mechanical ergogenic aids is to maximize any advantage that may be obtained from these external forces or to minimize any adverse resistance effects. For sports that depend on external forces for motion, such as sailing, some research efforts have focused on ways to harness those forces more effectively, such as the design of better sails. However, most of the research has focused on reducing the resistive effects of gravitational pull, decreasing air and water resistance, and favorably modifying frictional forces.

Gravitational Force

The most significant gravitational force acting upon you is exerted by the earth, which is constantly pulling your body downward. The magnitude of this effect depends basically on two factors. The first is your distance from the center of the earth: The closer you are, the greater is the gravitational pull. Thus, at high altitudes and at certain latitudes performance in some athletic events may be improved simply because of a lower gravitational force. The second factor is your body mass (weight), including the mass of any equipment or clothing on your body. The greater the combined mass of your body, clothing, and equipment, the greater the gravitational pull; thus, the greater the force you need to develop in order to overcome gravity.

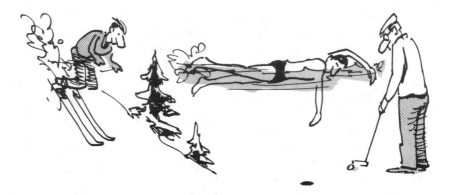

Gravity, buoyancy, and friction are three natural forces.

Fluid Resistance

Fluid resistance depends on a number of factors. One is the nature of the fluid. As all sports are performed in either air or water, these are the ones that concern us. Because air is less dense than water, the resistance of air is also less. We all know the difference in running in air versus water. However, certain environmental factors may change the density of these fluids. At high altitude the density of air is much less, so it creates less resistance to movement. This reduced air density, combined with a lower gravitational pull, may have contributed to the superior performances—including the phenomenal long jump of Bob Beamon—in the 1968 Olympic games in Mexico City, which has an altitude of approximately 7500 feet. Thus, in order to set personal records, athletes may desire to compete under certain environmental conditions, but the conditions would be the same for all athletes in the same competition.

Fluid resistance becomes of increasing concern for athletes who move at high speeds. Resistance in air and water increases disproportionately to the increase in velocity, or speed. In essence, resistance increases as the square of the velocity. Thus, doubling your running speed from 10 to 20 miles per hour will increase the resistance fourfold. This does not mean you have to increase your total energy production four times, for only part of the energy you produce is used to overcome air resistance; most of your energy is used to drive you forward by exerting force against the running surface. The point is, the amount of energy needed to over-come air resistance needs to be increased four times, not only twice (see Figure 7.1). Although the amount of energy needed to overcome this additional air resistance is not great at moderate running speeds, it is an important factor in high-speed sprints and becomes increasingly important at higher speeds, such as in bicycling and speed skating.

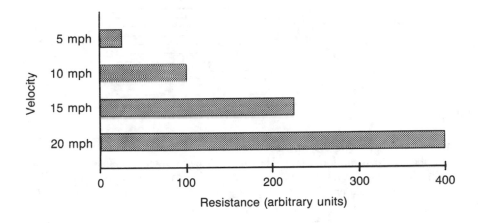

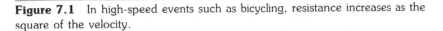

Figure 7.1   In high-speed events such as bicycling, resistance increases as the square of the velocity.

The resistance to motion in fluids is often called *drag*; two types of drag that interact with speed have important implications for sport. *Form drag* is the resistance created by the shape of the object moving through the fluid. As a child you probably put your hand out of the window of a moving car. If your fingers were pointed straight ahead your hand knifed through the air with little resistance and you had little trouble keeping your arm in place. But if you pointed your finger tips straight up, the force against your hand was great enough to pull your arm back. This is a perfect example of how the form of an object may influence air resistance (see Figure 7.2). *Surface drag* is a second type of resistance; its magnitude depends on the size and nature of the surface. In general, the larger and rougher the surface, the greater the drag.

There is little you can do about the greater air or water resistance that occurs naturally as you increase your speed in such sports as bicycling and swimming, but you may be able to reduce form and surface drag. Also, although not previously mentioned, there are other forces created when objects move through fluids, such as lift and spin effects, that may be important considerations in some sports.

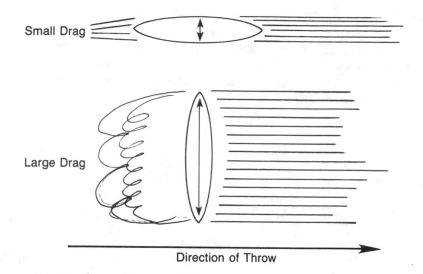

Small Drag

Large Drag

Direction of Throw

Figure 7.2 The larger the cross-sectional surface of an object to the oncoming fluid, the greater is the form drag. Thrown correctly, a discus will knife through the air with much less resistance than when it is thrown poorly. A poor release will create turbulence and considerable drag.

Frictional Resistance

Frictional resistance is similar to but different than fluid resistance. Whereas fluid resistance occurs between a solid object and a fluid, frictional resistance occurs between two solid objects in contact with each other, either while stationary or while moving. Both frictional and fluid resistance may be operative in the same sport. For example, a bicyclist is concerned not only with air resistance against both body and bicycle, but also with the frictional resistance created between the tires and the ground.

Friction represents resistance to movement. One test designed to measure the amount of frictional force between two solid objects is to place one object on top of the other on a flat surface, such as a small block of wood on a long plank, and then to slowly tilt the lower object. The angle at which the block begins to slide on the plank can be determined mathematically and provides a measure of the frictional force between these two objects. The greater the angle to which the plank must be lifted, the greater the frictional force between the two objects.

The magnitude of the frictional force between two solid objects depends primarily on two factors. One is the weight of one object that is perpendicular to the second one. Remember, gravity gives objects their weight and the force of gravity works perpendicularly towards the center of the earth. Let's use the example just described. As the plank is tilted, the force of gravity working on the block begins to deviate from the perpendicular so that less of the block weight is perpendicular to the plank surface, which causes the block to slide. In general, the greater the weight of the block, the greater the frictional force. The second factor influencing the frictional force is the nature of the surfaces of the two objects. If the surfaces of the block and the plank are both rough, the plank will have to be elevated to a steep angle before the block slides, which indicates a high frictional force. If the plank and the block are both smooth and polished, sliding will occur at a relatively small angle because there is little frictional force.

In sports, friction is a double-edged sword. Either too much or too little may impair performance. For example, a sprinter needs a certain amount of frictional resistance between her shoe and the track. Based on Newton's third law of motion, the action of her foot pushing downward and backward on the track surface results in a reaction of the track to push her upward and forward. If the friction between her shoe and the track is too low, possibly because her spikes are worn down or the track is worn smooth, her foot might slip and she will not get the maximal forward reaction desired. Conversely, spikes that are too long might increase the frictional forces excessively and also reduce speed.

There are also other mechanical forces or principles, such as *buoyancy* and *elasticity*, that may affect athletic performance. These will be incorporated in the discussion later, when appropriate.

General Applications
of Mechanical Ergogenic Aids

Unlike nutrition, physiology, pharmacology, and psychology, mechanics is an exact science, as it is based on proven laws of physics. For example, the theoretical values of many of the ergogenic aids discussed in previous chapters are still unsupported and need to be studied in rigorous research with athletes. This may be because individuals may respond differently to these ergogenic aids. If we give 300 milligrams of caffeine to 10 different subjects, the magnitude of the physiological responses may be different in every subject. However, if we change the form of a bicycle helmet and measure the change in air resistance in a wind tunnel, we can predict precisely how much energy will be saved by a bicyclist traveling at any speed.

Due to the exacting nature of the laws of physics, the development of mechanical ergogenic aids is often facilitated by the use of computers. All forces known to affect performance can be entered into the computer and manipulated in a variety of ways to predict the most optimal body position or equipment design. Thus, much of the research associated with the development of mechanical ergogenic aids is simply the application of laws of physics to sport. For example, Newton's second law of motion deals with the interrelationships of force, mass, and acceleration. In essence, *acceleration of an object is directly proportional to the force applied to it and inversely proportional to its mass.* All other things being equal, a given force will produce greater acceleration of a lighter object than a heavier one. As we shall see later, however, if all other things are not equal in relation to the factors affecting sports performance, some mechanical changes may not be beneficial.

Some of the recommendations in this chapter are based on theoretical values alone and not on actual research findings. Many of the improvements in athletic performance that may occur from using mechanical ergogenic aids may be so small that they cannot be detected in experimentation with humans because of normal day-to-day variation in performance. For example, wind-tunnel tests might show that a properly designed bicycle helmet could reduce air resistance enough to save 30 seconds in a 25-mile race. The mathematics of this conclusion based on laws of physics is beyond doubt, but, as the beneficial effect is so small, testing it in actual experimentation with humans in a 25-mile race might not be practical because variations in human physical performance may obscure this small effect. Yet, small as it is, 30 seconds could be the difference between victory and defeat.

On the other hand, there has been some human research supporting the ergogenic benefits of several mechanical aids. These findings will be used to support recommendations where relevant. The discussion in this chapter will focus on three general applications of mechanical ergogenic aids: biomechanics of the human body, sportswear, and sports equipment. There are potentially hundreds of different applications of mechanical ergogenic aids in these three areas, so a rather broad approach will be used when discussing the theoretical values, research findings, and recommendations in each area.

Human Body Biomechanics

Theoretical Basis

Just as the genes you inherited from your parents may provide you with physiological characteristics essential for success in athletics, they have also provided you with a unique set of morphological characteristics that may predispose you to success in some sports and limit your ability in others. Two important morphological characteristics are your height and the size, shape, and length of the bones in your skeleton. Taller individuals have a natural advantage in such sports as basketball and high jumping, whereas shorter individuals have similar advantages in sports such as gymnastics. Individuals with long arms may be more successful in throwing a discus; those with shorter arms may have an advantage in weight lifting. In female athletes, narrow hips may provide an advantage in sprint running.

Research conducted with athletes has revealed that certain body types, or *somatotypes*, tend to gravitate toward specific sports or positions in sports. For example, most elite distance runners have relatively lean body frames, most high jumpers are tall, and most interior linemen in professional football are large-boned and muscular. Even so, there is still a wide range of body types that may be successful in any given sport. Factors other than morphological characteristics may be more important in determining athletic success. Although your body type may limit your ability in certain sports, and although there is little you can do to change your height or bone structure, there are several biomechanical aspects of your body that you can change to possibly improve performance in some sports.

Sports Skills.   Theoretically, you have essentially two means of improving athletic performance through modification of your body biomechanics. First, you might be able to apply force to the desired movement in a more effective and efficient manner. Physiologically you may have highly developed human energy systems, but if that energy is not applied effectively performance will not be optimal. You could have a powerful lactic acid energy system that provides you the potential to be an excellent 100-meter swimmer, but if you do not have the necessary swimming skills much of this energy will be wasted as you thrash your way down the pool.

Body Position and Body Mass.   The second means of improving performance is to adjust your body biomechanics to modify the amount of resistance your body provides to movement. In high-speed sports, such as bicycling and speed skating, changing your body position can help to reduce air resistance. The proper position of a swimmer during various phases of the stroke can reduce water resistance. Decreasing your body weight can reduce the effect of gravitational pull and be helpful in such sports as gymnastics, where body weight needs to be supported. Increasing the body weight will increase friction and gravitational pull on the body and may be important for sumo wrestlers and interior linemen in football as a means of resisting movement.

Research Findings

Researchers in sport biomechanics are constantly looking for ways to improve athletic performance by modifying the ways that athletes apply their muscular forces to generate movement. Currently the United States Olympic

Committee (USOC) has a corps of sport biomechanists in major universities throughout the United States studying the movement patterns of elite athletes in a wide variety of sports. These researchers have at their disposal an array of advanced technological equipment to record and analyze human movement, including high-speed video cameras interfaced with computers to provide almost instantaneous analyses.

Biomechanics to Increase Force and Decrease Resistance.   One of the major thrusts of biomechanical research is to develop specific sports skills so that the athlete's energy forces are applied to movement in the most effective manner possible. Mechanical analyses of the arm pull in swimming and rowing, the leg and poling action in cross-country skiing, the sprint start in track, and the arm and leg movements in the high jump takeoff are just a few examples of the research that may provide more effective techniques of applying force. For example, the positions of the arms and hands in swimming the various strokes have been analyzed in order to provide the most effective surface area and angle during the pull phase, thus maximizing the application of force and providing the most beneficial lifting effect. Many of the results generated from this type of research have a general application to all athletes, but one of the advantages of modern computerized analyses is that they can adapt the skill to the individual athlete. At present, individual biomechanical skill analyses are done primarily with elite athletes, but eventually the technology may filter down to athletes at other levels of competition.

Depending on the sport, research involving wind-tunnel tests suggests that a change in the position or surface area of the body might help to decrease resistance to movement (see Figure 7.3). In high-speed sports such as bicycling, speed skating, downhill skiing, bobsledding, and luge, assuming a streamlined body position will help to decrease air resistance. In luge, the body is in nearly the ideal position with the feet leading the way and knifing through the air, similar to your hand out a car window with fingertips straight forward. In the other four sports the athlete attempts to curve the body into a rounded position similar to a teardrop. This teardrop position reduces form drag by minimizing the surface area of the body exposed to the wind and allowing the air to flow smoothly over the body, thus decreasing wind resistance. At high speeds such techniques become extremely important, for nearly 90 percent of the resistance to motion may be due to air resistance. Similar research techniques that measure resistance in swimmers while pulling them through water with a special apparatus reveals that the position of the body in the water, such as the orientation of the legs in the recovery phase of the breast stroke, may be modified to reduce form drag and water resistance.

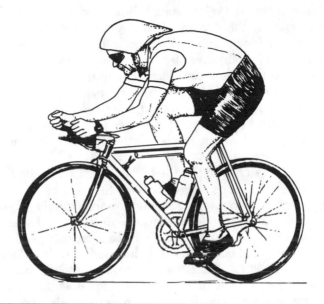

Figure 7.3   Modification of the body into a streamlined position will help reduce form drag.

Drafting.   Research has shown that other techniques can reduce air resistance and be effectively applied in some sports. At high speeds, the technique of *drafting* behind a bicyclist may demand about 30 percent less power output in the trailing rider. The lead rider takes the brunt of the air resistance and reduces the velocity of the wind, thus markedly decreasing air resistance on the trailing rider. Research also suggests that drafting may be beneficial in running, particularly in road races into a head wind. At average road-running speeds air resistance accounts for about 6 to 7 percent of the energy cost, but this percentage may increase markedly when you are running into a strong head wind. By tucking in behind a larger runner or a group of runners you will receive the benefit of less air resistance. In effect, drafting helps to save your energy for the latter stages of the race. The lead bicyclist or runner may be working at 80 percent of capacity, while the trailing athlete may be cruising at 70 percent or lower.

A technique used by swimmers to decrease water resistance is to shave the head and all other body hair in attempts to decrease surface drag. Although experimental research with swimmers has not validated the effectiveness of this procedure, the theoretical basis is sound. Creating a smoother skin surface could reduce surface drag.

Body Mass and Sports Performance.   Both theoretical considerations and research suggest that the composition of your body may significantly affect your performance in sports. Your body weight is composed of a variety of tissues, but for purposes of this discussion we will consider only two major components: body fat and lean body mass. Most of your lean body mass consists of muscle tissue, which is approximately 70 percent water. Thus, water can be considered a third component of your body weight. Although research has not revealed a specific percentage of body fat or lean body mass ideal for any given sport, it has provided enough data to make some generalities.

In general, research supports the finding that excess body fat may impair performance in sports where the body needs to be moved rapidly or efficiently, such as high jumping or long-distance running. Epidemiological research reveals low body-fat percentages in such athletes as distance runners, high jumpers, gymnasts, ballet dancers, sprinters, and others where excess body fat could be a disadvantage. Studies with children have revealed that those with higher levels of body fat are slower, have less agility, and cannot jump as far as leaner children. Experimental studies in which weights were strapped to the body of runners to simulate body fat demonstrated a decrease in efficiency when running. Such research findings in sport simply reflect the basic laws of physics; more energy is required to move a greater mass against the force of gravity. Although a certain amount of body fat is necessary for optimal health and physiological functioning, too much fat is simply excess baggage. For example, research involving physiological measurements has suggested that a 160-pound male runner can expect to improve performance by about 6 minutes in a 26.2-mile marathon if he loses 5 percent of his body weight, the equivalent of 8 pounds of fat.

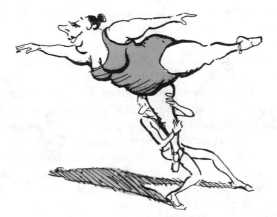

Excess body fat may be a disadvantage in many activities.

As many athletes do lose weight for competition, a number of research studies have studied the effects of different weight loss procedures on tests of physical performance. In general, rapid starvation and dehydration techniques to lose weight can result in serious impairment of performance, particularly endurance performance, because they deplete body-water stores and muscle and liver glycogen. Although body fat is lost with such techniques, so too is lean body mass, most notably muscle tissue. Consequently, other types of physical performance, such as strength and anaerobic endurance, may be affected adversely.

In sport events characterized by short bursts of power to move the body, such as high jumping, rapid loss of water weight through dehydration might benefit performance. A recent study noted an improvement in vertical jumping ability following an athlete's use of a diuretic to facilitate loss of body water. However, as noted in chapter 4, diuretics are drugs and their use in sports is banned by the International Olympic Committee (IOC).

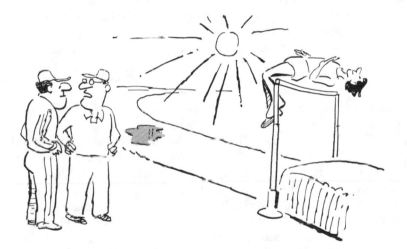

Weight loss through use of diuretics may benefit performance, but what an embarrassment!

Research has shown that slower weight losses achieved through exercise and moderate restriction of caloric intake will help to maintain performance capacity. Lean muscle mass may also be maintained by a properly designed weight-training program. Thus, a proper weight-reduction program can be very effective in improving performance in certain sports.

In some sports an increase in body weight may be an advantage. For example, in contact sports, such as football, ice hockey, and sumo wrestling, a greater body mass can help maintain stability and resist forces generated by opponents. However, although a little extra body fat might be useful in such sports, the increased body weight should be primarily in the form of muscle tissue. Research with professional football players, even many interior linemen, reveals relatively low levels of body fat. Moreover, literally hundreds of weight-training studies have shown that increases in muscle mass are usually accompanied by increases in strength, power, and performance.

Recommendations

As you probably realize, most of the methods to improve athletic performance through modification of body biomechanics are based on proper coaching and training. The development of the most efficient mechanical skills specific to a given sport, including how to maximize the application of force and minimize any resistant forces, occurs through sound analysis and the teaching of a knowledgeable coach. Training and nutrition are the keys to proper weight control, and sound programs can be obtained from coaches, sport nutritionists, and other sports medicine personnel. Remember—the use of such drugs as diuretics to decrease body weight rapidly is illegal.

Sport Skill Improvement.   The scope of this book does not allow for a detailed presentation of the biomechanics underlying the numerous skills found in sports. Some excellent books are available that cover sport biomechanics in general, whereas others focus on the biomechanics of a specific sport. *The Biomechanics of Sports Techniques* by James Hay is a prime example of the former, and *The Physiology and Biomechanics of Cycling* by Irvin Faria and Peter Cavanagh is an excellent example of the latter.

Elite performers are already functioning at a high level and may thus need only minor modifications in their styles. In such cases, high-speed filming and computer analysis by an expert in the field may be useful to detect any flaws and provide the basis for subsequent recommendations for improvement. Many coaches in colleges and high schools and numerous tennis and golf professionals also use high-speed video to improve the skills of their athletes. Such analyses may be a sound approach to enhance your skill performance. Analysis and feedback from a knowledgeable coach or professional can be invaluable.

A number of self-help resources are also available. As previously mentioned, books specific to a given sport may provide current information on proper skill development. Films and video tapes of selected sports skills are also commercially available.

Weight Control.   In any weight-control program, whether the object is to lose or gain weight, it is important to follow sound principles of nutrition. Again, the scope of this book does not allow for a detailed discussion of weight-control programs, but in general you should not lose more than 2 pounds per week unless under medical supervision. A deficit of 1000 calories per day will result in the loss of about 2 pounds per week; such a deficit may be achieved by expending 500 calories per day through exercise and decreasing food intake by 500 calories. The amount of exercise necessary to burn 500 calories is the approximate equivalent of running 5 miles. Simply reducing the amount of fat and sugar in your diet is usually all that is necessary to save 500 dietary calories per day.

To gain weight in the form of muscle mass requires a proper training program with weights, such as free weights or Nautilus, and the intake of an additional 400 to 500 calories daily. A gain of about one pound per week appears to be a realistic goal on such a program. Consult your physician or a local nutritionist to recommend sensible programs for weight control.

Sportswear

Theoretical Basis

Required for all sports is some type of uniform, ranging from the brief suit of the male swimmer to the full wardrobe of the downhill skier. Wearing apparel designed specifically for athletes may serve a variety of purposes, one of the most important being protection from the elements or from injury. Special fabrics enable runners to keep warm and dry while training in wet, cold conditions, modern running shoes are designed to balance cushioning and motion control to help prevent overuse injuries, and helmets may prevent serious injury to the head during accidents in high-speed and collision sports.

The type of sportswear an athlete selects or is required to wear may also affect performance. Virtually everything athletes wear in competition has been modified in some way in attempts to improve performance. Helmets, glasses, uniforms, gloves, socks, and shoes have been engineered to save minutes, seconds, and even thousandths of a second in athletic competition. Sportswear providing a competitive edge over an opponent may be considered ergogenic.

The design of sportswear for ergogenic purposes is based on the same principles of physics underlying modification of body biomechanics to improve performance. Depending on the sport, sportswear may be engineered to decrease air resistance, water resistance, and gravitational forces, to increase or decrease friction, or to increase buoyancy. Theoretically, such effects could enhance athletic performance.

Research Findings

Wind Resistance.   Research conducted in wind-tunnel tests conclusively shows that if specially designed sportswear can reduce form drag or surface drag compared to traditional sportswear, then air resistance or water resistance will be reduced correspondingly. In high-speed sports like downhill skiing, speed skating, and bicycling, everything the athlete wears has been streamlined to make it more aerodynamic. As mentioned earlier, based on energy savings, use of an aerodynamic helmet in bicycling may save up to 30 seconds in a 25-mile race. Streamlining the boots in downhill skiing may provide an advantage of less than a second, but that second could be the critical difference. The use of full-length, skintight uniforms may help decrease air resistance at high speeds by 6 to 10 percent, which might permit a 4000-meter pursuit bicyclist to go three seconds faster. Form-fitting swimsuits, especially for females, have similar effects on water resistance.

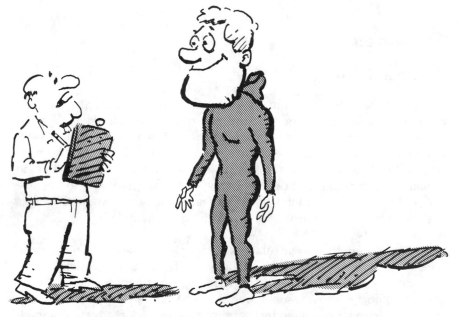

"Well, we got your body down to the right size. Now we have to do something about your head."

For runners, Figure 7.4 illustrates the increase in *aerodynamic drag* with different types of clothing or hair length. Although only a few world-class track sprinters, who may reach speeds over 25 miles per hour in a 100-meter dash, have experimented with skintight uniforms, that may soon change. Some recent research from Simon Fraser University in Canada has suggested that the use of a full uniform, including a hood, made of a new

Japanese material similar to Saran Wrap, could improve the world record in the 100-meter dash by 0.17 seconds. The lead investigator also noted that such a uniform could be useful to distance runners as well, possibly improving the mile record by 3 seconds.

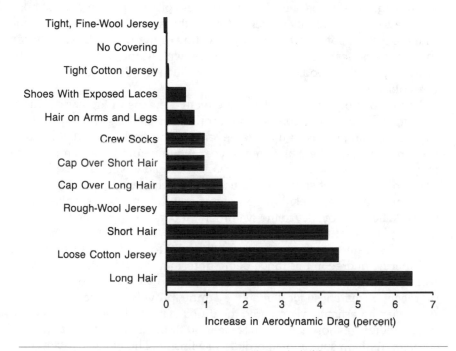

Figure 7.4 Aerodynamic effect of various kinds of clothing on a runner is charted. The wool jersey ranks ahead of no covering because it functions like the dimples on a golf ball to reduce air resistance. *Note.* From "Athletic Clothing" by Chester Kyle. Copyright © 1986 by Scientific American, Inc. All rights reserved. Reprinted by permission.

As noted before, it is often difficult to verify the theoretical benefits of mechanical ergogenic aids in actual human athletic competition because some of the improvements are so small that they may be clouded over by the normal daily variations in human physical performance. However, the 1968 Olympic games in Mexico City provided an unusual opportunity to study the effects of reduced air resistance on performance in speed events by large numbers of elite athletes. In general, there was a 1.7 percent improvement by sprinters.

Buoyancy. An improved buoyancy would be advantageous to swimmers because their higher body position in the water could reduce water resistance since more of their body could move through air. In addition, less energy would have to be expended to keep the body from sinking. Although increasing your body-fat percentage will increase your buoyancy, this procedure is not usually recommended for swimmers. It is interesting, however, that when the performances of males and females are compared in a variety of sports, the performance of the females comes closest to the males in swimming, possibly because females possess greater percentages of body fat due to hormonal differences between the sexes. It is also interesting that the first person to swim the frigid waters of the Bering Strait between the United States and Russia was a female with 40 percent body fat. The body fat provided good buoyancy and the much-needed insulation against the cold water.

There does not appear to be any effective means of increasing buoyancy in most swimming competition, for flotation devices are illegal. However, swimming is one of the three events in the traditional triathlon and triathlons are often held at a time of year when a cold water temperature may subject an athlete to hypothermia, or a rapid lowering of body temperature. Thus, wet suits may be used by triathletes in order to prevent hypothermia (excessively low body temperature), but wet suits also provide additional buoyancy to the swimmer. At present, in competition under the jurisdiction of the Triathlon Federation USA, wet suits may be worn only if the water temperature is lower than 70 to 74 degrees Fahrenheit, the specific degree in this range being determined by the race director. If wet suits are permitted it may be a good idea to wear one, for the results of recent research suggest that they may provide ergogenic benefits. Australian investigators compared the times of trained swimmers covering 1,500 meters, almost a mile, while wearing three different suits: a wet suit, a Lycra triathlon suit, and an ordinary swimsuit. The athletes' swim times while wearing the wet suits were significantly faster than when wearing the other two suits, presumably due to the wet suit's buoyancy effect.

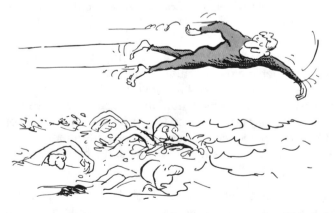

"I think the design of these wet suits to increase buoyancy is getting a little out of hand."

Sportswear Weight.   The weight of sportswear can impair performance in some sports because more energy is required to overcome the additional gravitational force. Thus, designers of athletic apparel have used modern fabrics and materials to provide the lightest sportswear possible. Although almost all sportswear has benefited from such research and design, sports shoes have received considerable attention.

The running boom triggered tremendous interest in shoe research. With hundreds of millions of dollars in sales at stake, many shoe companies developed their own engineering research labs to design a better running shoe than their competition. Many of these companies sponsored racing teams composed of international class runners; some of their labs employed sport biomechanists and exercise physiologists to help research and design the optimal racing shoe for these elite runners.

Any savings in weight of the running shoe should be an advantage when an athlete must move rapidly or over a long period of time. Several research studies have supported this point. In one study, runners ran on a treadmill at a set speed wearing shoes of different weights while their oxygen consumption was measured. As expected, while wearing heavier shoes the runners' oxygen uptake was higher, which indicates that more energy was required than when the runners wore lighter shoes. The projected savings in energy amount to about 0.28 percent for each ounce, so when a 5-ounce racing flat is substituted for a 10-ounce training shoe, the savings could amount to several minutes in long-distance running.

Sportswear Composition.   Some preliminary research has also suggested that the composition of the shoe might provide an ergogenic effect. Shoe manufacturers use materials with different amounts of elasticity to absorb the force of the foot's impact with the ground. The midsole of the shoe compresses on contact and acts as a kind of shock absorber, providing cushioning as the foot lands. Due to the midsole's elasticity, as it resumes its original shape some of the compression forces stored in it may help increase foot speed as the rebound forces return to the foot of the runner. Several studies with elite distance runners, similar in design to the studies with shoe weight, have suggested that a midsole composed of encased air may provide an ergogenic effect that shoes with conventional midsoles do not supply.

Although the weight and composition of a shoe may be important factors in selecting a pair for competition, any possible gain due to a lower weight or air sole may be lost if the motion of the foot is not controlled. Improper foot plant or excessive rolling of the foot can waste energy that could be used for forward propulsion.

Sports shoes may also be designed to provide the optimal amount of friction for a given sport. A bicyclist wants a shoe with maximal friction between foot and pedal in order to decrease slipping during a race, whereas a bowler desires a smooth sole to minimize friction on the sliding foot during delivery of the ball. Depending on the needs of the athlete, shoes have been customized to optimize frictional forces. Thus, the soles of some shoes may be designed to prevent slipping but also contain small smooth spots near the base of the toes to allow for quick pivots, such as in tennis and wrestling. One interesting research project was the application of high-speed filming with sprinters to improve the track shoe. The filming revealed that the foot of sprinters rolls inward as it lands and the lateral outside part of the foot comes into contact with the surface. If this surface is smooth, possible slipping can occur as the sprinter drives forward. Thus, a section of rough material is incorporated in the lateral portion of the shoe to help increase frictional forces. This change is relatively minor but could make the difference in an extremely close race.

Recommendations

It appears obvious that appropriate sportswear can improve performance. Serious competitive athletes should stay abreast of modern technological developments and research findings regarding the application of sportswear modification to their sport. Many of these applications are reported in popular journals that are available for almost every sport.

Most athletes competing at the elite level are already benefiting from technological advances in sportswear design. The companies or countries that sponsor them see to it that they have the best apparel available, for it is to their economic or political benefit. In fact, some sportswear is customized to the special biomechanical needs of the individual athlete.

For athletes at other levels of competition where sportswear can make a difference, the basic recommendation is to select apparel that is supported by sound theory and research. If air or water resistance may hamper performance, avoid the use of loose clothing or other apparel that would increase this resistance. Select sportswear designed to make you more streamlined and aerodynamic. To reduce the effects of gravitational forces select shoes and other apparel that are lightweight, as long as they still function effectively.

Proper sportswear can be a very effective ergogenic aid. However, if all athletes have it, then there is no competitive edge. This is usually the case in national and international competition, but may not be so at lower levels.

Sports Equipment

Theoretical Basis

For the purpose of this discussion, sports equipment is differentiated from sportswear. We shall consider sports equipment as any ball, instrument, or vehicle essential to the conduct of the sport. One of the basic premises of sport is that an equipment advantage should not be instrumental in deciding the outcome of the contest. In some sports this is no problem, as basically no equipment is used. In swimming, distance running, and wrestling, for instance, the competition is strictly between the athletes. In other sports, however, equipment is crucial to the outcome and a superior design may provide an advantage. You may recall that in the 1984 Winter Olympics the United States bobsled team rushed around in the last few days prior to competition trying to buy one of the newly designed European sleds. Or you might remember when, in the 1984 Summer Olympics, the American team appeared with their futuristic bicycles. Were the Americans the beneficiaries of modern sport technology in the summer, but at a disadvantage in the winter?

High Technology in Sports.   In attempts to make competition equal between participating athletes, all sports have rules governing various aspects of sports equipment, such as weight, dimensions, and design. Whereas design engineers can do little to improve some equipment—such as the 16-pound shot, which is not very aerodynamic—they can make remarkable changes in others that will improve performance. For example, older rules for the javelin basically stipulated its weight and length but said little of its design. Consequently, engineers designed an aerodynamic javelin that could be thrown well beyond 300 feet, which in some places of competition put it in the stands with the spectators, many of whom did not consider this a good example of a spectator sport. Subsequently, the rules were changed to include limitations on the design of the javelin.

One of the most interesting accounts concerning sports equipment technology was the cover story in the August 1987 issue of *Scientific American* about the Stars and Stripes, the United States' entry in the America's Cup international sailing competition for 12-meter yachts. In 1983, following the first loss ever for the United States since the America's Cup competition began, a syndicate was formed to win back the Cup by applying the best American technology available to the design of the yacht. The engineers were constrained by the 12-Meter Rule, which basically represents a limit on the combination of hull measurements and sail dimensions. However, the designers can make some tradeoffs, such as choosing a longer hull and compensating with a smaller sail area. The article documents how engineers used modern computer technology to design the boat within the 12-Meter Rule to meet the challenges of sailing under different weather conditions.

One of the interesting points in this article was that the America's Cup represented competition not only between sailors, but also between the technologists of the different countries involved. Highly skilled sailors are needed, but if the boat is not on the leading edge of technology then the sailors, no matter how skilled, are at a substantial disadvantage. This problem does not exist in Olympic sailing because all competitors use boats of the same design. However, in other sports there is some leeway in the design of the equipment so sport technologists may be able to provide athletes with a competitive advantage. You may be as well trained a triathlete as the individual next to you, but if you show up with your old Columbia one-speed with balloon tires and he or she has a $5,000 customized Italian model, between the two of you it's a pretty safe bet who will win the bike phase of the competition.

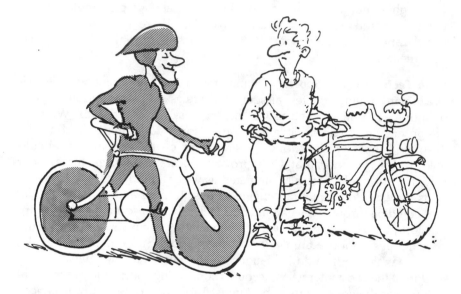

The advent of computer-assisted design (CAD) has completely transformed the process of designing sports equipment. Because the mathematical laws of physics are immutable, numerous variables such as weight, size, wind velocity, and others may be entered into a computer program and manipulated until optimal results are obtained. As the results are totally predictable, the computer easily handles changes in any variable. On the other hand, the older techniques required the actual production of a prototype model for testing. Taking as an example the Stars and Stripes, a computer run to test the variables would cost about 15 dollars, whereas production of a prototype would cost nearly a million dollars, and take much more time.

Ergogenic Aspects of Sports Equipment.   Although sports equipment may be designed for a variety of purposes, such as comfort and safety, from an ergogenic standpoint the major purpose is to improve athletic performance. Changes in design depend on the needs of the athlete. For example, the size and elastic characteristics of balls can be manipulated to make them travel faster or slower when struck. In baseball, a batter usually prefers a livelier ball for it will rebound faster and produce more hits. On the other hand, the pitcher and fielders prefer a less lively ball for opposite reasons.

It is interesting to note that the economics of sports demographics may influence the design of sports equipment. For example, many of the baby-boom generation who flocked to the tennis courts in the 1960s have stopped playing, possibly because age has slowed their reaction time and performance has deteriorated. In an attempt to attract older players back to the sport, manufacturers have designed some tennis balls to travel slower when hit, giving the player more time to react.

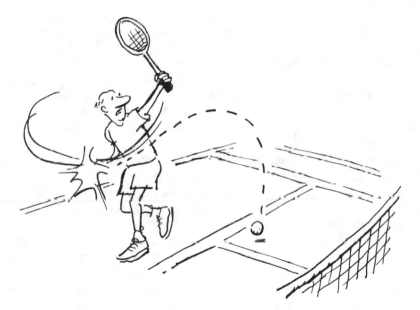

"I think they have slowed these balls down a little too much."

There are several basic categories of equipment used in sports. Objects are designed to be propelled for distance or accuracy, such as balls, javelins, and arrows. Implements are used to receive objects and to impart or control the application of force to objects, such as tennis rackets, lacrosse sticks, and bows. Other equipment serves to transport the athlete; in some cases the athlete provides the majority of the force for movement, such as to bicycles and cross-country skis, whereas in other cases the athlete is primarily responsible for controlling a vehicle, such as a bobsled or a sailboat, whose movement is produced by the forces of gravity or wind. A major goal of engineers is to improve the effectiveness of the various types of sports equipment to optimally fulfill their basic functions.

Research Findings

Several different research techniques have been used to improve equipment design. As previously mentioned, CAD can be used effectively in the design of almost any equipment. Wind-tunnel tests to measure air and water resistance have been used when these forces might be modified to improve speed, height, or distance. The impact forces between balls and striking implements have been studied directly, for example, by applying a known force to a ball to see how fast and far the ball will travel after impact.

The results of such research have led to significant improvements in athletic performance. One glaring example is the advent of the fiberglass pole used in pole vaulting. Vaulters using aluminum poles tried for years to break the elusive barrier of 15 feet and finally succeeded. However, immediately after the fiberglass pole became available vaulters began easily scaling this former barrier, and the world record is now approaching 20 feet. With improving technology pole vaulters may have to learn sky diving in order to land safely.

Research engineers interested in improving sports equipment must work within the limits of the rules governing equipment for any given sport. However, when engineers are too successful, many of the sport-governing bodies impose additional rules and restrictions, as noted previously in the case of javelin design.

There are literally hundreds of examples that could be cited to illustrate the point that technological modifications in equipment can improve athletic performance. The scope of this book does not allow for such a lengthy discussion of specific research studies. Thus, only several general applications will be noted below.

Sports Objects.   If the purpose of a sport is to propel an object for distance or accuracy, then the object itself may be modified to achieve these objectives. As noted before, the size and composition of balls can affect their speed, and hence distance. You may recall the Superball of years ago. Can you imagine playing handball or squash with it? The design of the object may also affect distance and accuracy. The distance the javelin could be thrown was improved markedly by adding a flattened tail section that improved its aerodynamics by providing a greater lifting effect. As another example, the number and configuration of the dimples in a golf ball can be manipulated to drastically reduce air resistance, thus improving distance. One golf ball design even had a built-in gyroscope to reduce the magnitude of the curve and improve accuracy. Unfortunately for habitual hookers, this type of ball was banned. A similar design has also been used with American footballs, permitting a perfect spiral on every pass.

Sports Implements.   Sports implements used to impart movement to objects have also received much research attention. The size and composition of the implement may influence its striking characteristics. Some research has shown that an aluminum bat may impart more speed to a baseball than a wooden bat. This finding was attributed to the uniform distribution of material in the hollow aluminum bat compared to a less uniform density in the wooden bat. In essence, the more uniform composition provided a more effective center of percussion, resulting in less vibration or wasted energy on impact and hence more speed; the *center of percussion* is also the so-called *sweet spot*. One of the advantages of the larger heads in tennis rackets is the increased sweet spot. Golf clubs and other striking implements can also be designed along these lines.

Sports Vehicles.   Engineers have significantly improved the mechanics of sports equipment used to move the athlete, such as the bobsled, luge, sailboat, bicycle, and skis. Most of the research has focused on means of reducing resistance, either fluid or frictional. Modifications in the design of the bicycle illustrate how decreasing resistance can improve performance. An elite competitor's bicycle is lightweight due to special metal alloys, is aerodynamically designed from the seat down to the water bottle, is equipped with wheels and tires specifically designed to minimize air and rolling resistance, and may be tailored to the specific body configurations of the cyclist. The bicycles used by the successful American cyclists in the 1984 Olympics were the result of modern sport technology.

Recommendations

Our general recommendation regarding sports equipment is comparable to the one we offered on the use of sportswear: You need to be aware of changes in equipment design brought about by research and technology. Again, popular magazines for specific sports often reveal such advancements that appear to be supported by sound logic and research.

Elite athletes need to be assured that they have the best equipment available. If not, they will be at a definite mechanical disadvantage and a possible psychological disadvantage (if they know their opponents have better equipment). Although equipment disparity is not usually that great at this level of competition, there have been situations where it could make the difference between winning and losing.

For the everyday athlete, training is still the key to improved performance. However, if you are a serious competitor and want to be all that you can possibly be, then you can buy speed. How much you can buy depends on the size of your wallet. As a competitive bicyclist, you can buy a little speed with $60 bullhorn handlebars, a little more speed with lightweight wheels and sew-up tires for $500, and even more with a $5,000 aerodynamic bicycle. Eventually though, you reach a limit and training once again becomes the critical variable.

Legal and Ethical Considerations.   You need to be aware of the rules governing the use of such equipment in competition. For example, certain modifications in bicycles, such as wheel covers, may not be allowed in events sponsored by the Triathlon Federation USA.

It is to be assumed that research engineers and sport biomechanists will continue to search for ways to improve performance through the design of better equipment that conforms to the rules of competition. For example, bicycles designed to seat the cyclist in a recumbent position may reach speeds of 60 miles per hour. However, these recumbent bicycles are not allowed in competition. From an ethical viewpoint it is to be hoped that if sports equipment can make the difference in the outcome of competition then it should be available to *all* competing athletes.

Selected Readings

Books

Burke, E. (Ed.). (1986). *Science of cycling.* Champaign, IL: Human Kinetics.

Dyson, G. (1977). *The mechanics of athletics.* New York: Holmes and Meier.

Faria, I., & Cavanagh, P. (1978). *The physiology and biomechanics of cycling.* New York: Wiley.

Frederick, E. (Ed.). (1984). *Sport shoes and playing surfaces.* Champaign, IL: Human Kinetics.

Hay, J. (1978). *The biomechanics of sports techniques.* Englewood Cliffs, NJ: Prentice Hall.

Hay, J., & Reid, J. (1982). *The anatomical and mechanical bases of human motion.* Englewood Cliffs, NJ: Prentice Hall.

Nigg, B. (Ed.). (1986). *Biomechanics of running shoes.* Champaign, IL: Human Kinetics.

Reviews

Cavanagh, P., & Kram, R. (1985). Mechanical and muscular factors affecting the efficiency of human movement. *Medicine and Science in Sports and Exercise*, **17**, 326-331.

Frederick, E. (1983). Extrinsic biomechanical aids. In M. Williams (Ed.), *Ergogenic aids in sport* (pp. 323-339). Champaign, IL: Human Kinetics.

Frederick, E. (1987). No sweat. *Runner's World*, **22**, 78-83.

Gonzalez, R. (1987). Biophysical and physiological integration of proper clothing for exercise. *Exercise and Sport Sciences Reviews*, **15**, 261-295.

Kyle, C. (1986). Athletic clothing. *Scientific American*, **254**, 104-110.

Letcher, J., Marshall, J., Oliver, J., & Salvesen, N. (1987). Stars & Stripes. *Scientific American*, **257**, 34-40.

Lowdon, B., McKenzie, D., & Ridge, B. (1987). Effect of clothing and water temperature on triathlon swim performance. *Medicine and Science in Sports and Exercise*, **19**, S26.

Vaughan, C. (1984). Computer simulation of human motion in sports biomechanics. *Exercise and Sport Sciences Reviews*, **12**, 373-416.

Viitasalo, J., Kyrolainen, H., Bosco, C., & Alen, M. (1987). Effects of rapid weight reduction on force production and vertical jumping height. *International Journal of Sports Medicine*, **8**, 281-285.

Williams, K. (1985). The relationship between mechanical and physiological energy estimates. *Medicine and Science in Sports and Exercise*, **17**, 317-325.

Epilogue

AS INDICATED IN CHAPTER 1, the two primary factors that determine your ability to succeed in sports are your genetic endowment specific to a given physical or physiological characteristic and how well you train that characteristic. For example, to be a very successful endurance athlete you will need to have inherited the potential for a high maximal oxygen uptake from your parents, but you will also need to train hard in order to realize that potential. For your given genetic endowment and your current state of training, certain ergogenic aids may help to optimize your performance.

This book has been an attempt to provide basic coverage of most of the ergogenic aids that have been or are being used by athletes in attempts to improve performance. As you have probably observed, the available research reveals some significant differences between the various ergogenic aids relative to their ability to improve physical performance.

Research substantiates the ability of some aids, such as oxygen utilization during exercise or blood doping, to improve performance in endurance type events. With other aids, such as alkaline salts and phosphate salts, the research findings are rather mixed; a number of studies support their effectiveness to improve performance, whereas other studies find them ineffective. And finally with some aids, such as bee pollen and vitamin B_{15}, the available well-controlled research strongly suggests they do not improve physical performance.

Sport scientists will continue to explore possible ergogenic aids as legitimate means of improving performance. Sport biomechanists will attempt to improve skill efficiency; sport physiologists will experiment with new, sophisticated training methods; sport nutritionists will search for the optimal fuel; and sport psychologists will continue to refine their mental intervention techniques. Although the use of most drugs in sport is illegal, it is likely that some pharmacologists will conduct experiments on the effects of new agents on performance, and possibly find ones that cannot be detected by current testing methods.

With the increasing importance of sport in our society and the emphasis placed on winning, there is no doubt that there will be a wave of new ergogenic aids in the future. Much of the research may focus on individualized approaches and modification of the genetic potential.

Just as physical training for the elite athlete has become highly individualized, such an approach may also be utilized with ergogenic aids in the future. Let us look at caffeine as an example. Research has suggested that certain dosages of caffeine may be more effective than others as a means of improving performance. On the other hand, in some of the studies certain individuals actually experienced adverse reactions to caffeine. It is thus possible that certain ergogenic aids will have to be tailored specifically to meet the needs of the individual athlete. With the application of high technology to the sports sciences, such a situation may become very practical.

Genetic engineering may be the ultimate ergogenic aid. Through the manipulation of the genes that carry desirable physical or physiological characteristics, medical scientists may literally be able to create the superathlete. Although such an idea seems farfetched, some of you may recall the attempt by Adolph Hitler to create the superman race, the Aryans, by the more basic technique of pairing males and females who possessed the desired Aryan characteristics.

The technology of genetic engineering is available. Given the apparent political value assigned to sport by major international powers (some countries may interpret a victory in the Olympic Games as a reflection of the superiority of their political system), it might be only a matter of time before genetic engineering is applied to sports performance.

Appendix

Banned Ergogenic Aids

THE FOLLOWING LIST is a compilation of the major classes of ergogenic aids, with a *partial* listing of specific agents, that are banned for use
by athletes who participate in competition under the auspices of the International Olympic Committee (IOC), the United States Olympic Committee
(USOC), or the National Collegiate Athletic Association (NCAA). There
may be some slight variations in the major classes or specific agents between the different athletic-governing bodies, so *the athlete is advised to
consult the appropriate agency to determine the legality of any specific
medication or technique.*

PSYCHOMOTOR STIMULANT DRUGS

Amphetamine	Methylamphetamine
Benzphetamine	Norpseudoephedrine
Chlorphentermine	Pemoline
Cocaine	Phendimetrazine
Diethylpropion	Phenmetrazine
Dimethylamphetamine	Phentermine
Ethylamphetamine	Pipradrol
Fencamfamine	Prolintane
Meclofenoxate	Related compounds

CENTRAL NERVOUS SYSTEM STIMULANTS

Amiphenazole	Nikethamide
Bemegride	Picrotoxin
Doxapram	Strychnine
Ethamivan	Related compounds, for example,
Leptazol	caffeine; greater than 15 micrograms/milliliter urine

SYMPATHOMIMETIC AMINES

Clorprenaline

Ephedrine

Etafedreine

Isoetharine

Isoprenaline

Isoproterenol

Metaproterenol

Methoxyphenamine

Methylephedrine

Related compounds

OVER-THE-COUNTER DRUGS FOR COLDS AND SINUS INFECTIONS

Ephedrine

Phenylephrine

Phenylpropanolamine (and
   related cold products)

Propylhexedrine

Pseudoephedrine

NARCOTIC ANALGESICS

Anileridine

Codeine

Dextromoramide

Dihydrocodeine

Dipipanone

Ethylmorphine

Heroin

Hydrocodone

Hydromorphone

Levorphanol

Methadone

Morphine

Naloxone

Oxycodone

Pentazocine

Pethidine

Phenazocine

Piminodine

Thebacon

Trimerperidine

Related compounds

ANABOLIC STEROIDS

Clostebol

Danazol

Fluoxymesterone

Mesterolone

Metenolone

Methandienone

Methyltestosterone

Nandrolone (19-Nortestosterone)

Norethandrolone

Oxandrolone

Oxymesterone

Oxymetholone

Stanozolol

Testosterone (if the ratio of the
   total testosterone to that of
   epitestosterone in the urine
   is more than 6)

Related compounds

DIURETICS

Bendroflumethiazide

Benzthiazide

Bumetanide

Chlorothiazide

Chlorthalidone

Cyclothiazide

Ethacrynic Acid

Flumethiazide

Furosemide

Hydrochlorothiazide

Hydroflumethiazide

Metolazone

Polythiazide

Quinethazone

Spironolactone

Triamterene

Trichlormethiazide

Related compounds

SUBSTANCES BANNED FOR SPECIFIC SPORTS

Alcohol

Atenolol

Beta-blockers

Propranolol

Related compounds

STREET DRUGS

Heroin

Marijuana

THC (tetrahydrocannabinol)

Others

BLOOD DOPING

OTHER AGENTS

The use of certain drugs, such as local anesthetics, various asthma medications, and corticosteroids, may be banned or exempt from the banned list, depending on the circumstances. Consult with the appropriate athletic-governing authority.

Index

Fructose, 12, 41-42, 45, 46, 53
FT muscle fibers, 18, 20, 22, 23, 29, 30, 43, 44
    relation to lactic acid system, 25
Furosemide, 197

G

Gastric emptying, 46
Gastrointestinal distress. *See also* Diarrhea
    relation to alkaline salts, 130
    relation to carbohydrate intake, 50, 52
    relation to glucose polymers, 46
Gatorade, 75
Gelatin, 76
Genetic engineering, 3, 194
Genetics, relation to athletic performance, 193
Ginseng, 76
Girdano, D., 161
Glucose, 25, 41-42, 45. *See also* Carbohydrates
    ingestion of, 46
    relation to fatigue, 32, 44
    relation to oxygen system, 21
    relation to water intake, 75
Glucose-alanine cycle, 62
Glucose polymers, 42, 45, 46, 47, 52, 53
    relation to gastrointestinal distress, 46
    relation to water intake, 75
Glycerol, 54
Glycogen, 32, 41, 42, 43
    depletion and fatigue, 44
    loading. *See* Carbohydrates, loading of
    relation to lactic acid system, 20
    relation to oxygen system, 21
    supercompensation. *See* Carbohydrates, loading of
Glycogen-sparing theory, relation to caffeine, 89
Glycolysis, 20
Goal setting, 145, 147-148
Gout, 62
Gravitational forces, 167-168
Growth hormone. *See* hGH
Gymnasts
    use of diuretics by, 96
    vitamin intake of, 67

H

Haas, R., 122
Hay, J., 178
HCG, 101
HDL-C, effect of anabolic steroids on, 104
HDL-cholesterol. *See* HDL-C
Heart disease. *See* Coronary heart disease

About the Author

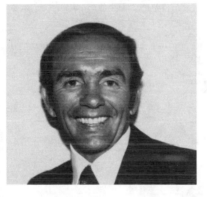

Dr. Williams earned a PhD in physical education and exercise science from the University of Maryland. He is director of the Human Performance Laboratory and the Wellness Institute and Research Center at Old Dominion University in Norfolk, Virginia.

In more than 20 years of research into ergogenic aids, Dr. Williams has earned numerous awards, honors, and grants. Two of the awards to his credit are the Outstanding Research Award from Old Dominion University and the prestigious Sarah and Rufus Tonelson Award for Teaching, Research, and Service Excellence.

Dr. Williams's personal experiences with ergogenic aids as a college athlete, a marathoner, an ultramarathoner, a triathlete, and a coach have given him unique insight into this emotionally charged issue. Dr. Williams is the editor of *Ergogenic Aids in Sport*, as well as the author of eight other books and dozens of articles. In his spare time, he enjoys skiing and running.